..........................

**Guide to Paediatric Clinical Research**

# Guide to
# Paediatric Clinical Research

Editors

*Klaus Rose*  Basel

*John N. van den Anker*  Washington, D.C./Rotterdam

8 figures and 8 tables, 2007

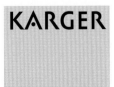

Basel · Freiburg · Paris · London · New York
Bangalore · Bangkok · Singapore · Tokyo · Sydney

**Klaus Rose**
Head Pediatrics
F. Hoffmann-La Roche Ltd.
Pharmaceuticals Division
Basel, Switzerland

**John N. van den Anker**
Division of Pediatric Clinical Pharmacology
Children's National Medical Center, and
Departments of Pediatrics, Pharmacology and
Physiology
George Washington University School of
Medicine and Health Sciences
Washington, D.C., USA
and
Department of Pediatrics
Erasmus MC-Sophia Children's Hospital
Rotterdam, The Netherlands

Library of Congress Cataloging-in-Publication Data

Guide to paediatric clinical research / editors, Klaus Rose, John N. van den
Anker.
   p. ; cm.
 Includes bibliographical references and index.
 ISBN-13: 978-3-8055-8201-8 (hard cover : alk. paper)
 ISBN-10: 3-8055-8201-3 (hard cover : alk. paper)
 1. Pediatrics--Research. 2. Clinical medicine--Research. 3.
Children--Research--Moral and ethical aspects. I. Rose, Klaus, 1953- II.
Van den Anker, John N.
 [DNLM: 1. Pediatrics. 2. Research Design. 3. Clinical
Trials--standards. 4. Drug Evaluation--methods. 5. Ethics, Research. 6.
Risk Assessment. WS 20 G946 2007]
 RJ85.G85 2007
 618.92--dc22
                        2006031666

Bibliographic Indices. This publication is listed in bibliographic services, including Current Contents® and Index Medicus.

Disclaimer. The statements, options and data contained in this publication are solely those of the individual authors and contributors and not of the publisher and the editor(s). The appearance of advertisements in the book is not a warranty, endorsement, or approval of the products or services advertised or of their effectiveness, quality or safety. The publisher and the editor(s) disclaim responsibility for any injury to persons or property resulting from any ideas, methods, instructions or products referred to in the content or advertisements.

Drug Dosage. The authors and the publisher have exerted every effort to ensure that drug selection and dosage set forth in this text are in accord with current recommendations and practice at the time of publication. However, in view of ongoing research, changes in government regulations, and the constant flow of information relating to drug therapy and drug reactions, the reader is urged to check the package insert for each drug for any change in indications and dosage and for added warnings and precautions. This is particularly important when the recommended agent is a new and/or infrequently employed drug.

© Copyright 2007 by S. Karger AG, P.O. Box, CH–4009 Basel (Switzerland)
www.karger.com
Printed in Switzerland on acid-free paper by Reinhardt Druck, Basel
ISBN-10: 3-8055–8201–3
ISBN-13: 978–3–8055–8201–8

# Contents

V

# Introduction from the Editors

Developing medicines for children is like designing a bridge to connect two different worlds – the very intimate world of parents taking care of their sick child and the complex world of an innovative pharmaceutical industry creating modern drugs. Drug development in general is already a complex process involving clinicians, regulatory authorities and pharmaceutical companies, but paediatric drug development adds another dimension to this complexity. Many more players have become intensively involved including governments that have become active to promote paediatric research, paediatric professional organisations that lobbied for these governmental actions, patients' and parents' organisations, and others.

Klaus Rose, chairman of the EFGCP Children's Medicines Working Party (www.efgcp.be) was approached at the end of 2005 by Karger publishers with the proposal to produce a short textbook on paediatric clinical trials. This proposal was welcomed by the members of the working party. John N. van den Anker, President of the European Society for Developmental, Perinatal and Paediatric Pharmacology (ESDP) for 2006 to 2008, volunteered to serve as co-editor.

The EFGCP is a forum that fosters strategic dialogue across the barriers of affiliations that are involved in clinical research. The Children's Medicines Working Party is composed of academic paediatricians, regulators, patients' advocacy groups, and pharmaceutical industry. Although this book is not an official EFGCP publication, the original nucleus of its emergence should be mentioned. All articles represent the authors' personal opinion, not the opinion of their respective affiliations.

Many areas are covered in these pages by authors from very different backgrounds. Authors' short biographies and their e-mail addresses are given in a separate listing. Feedback and comments are welcome and can be directed to the editors or to the individual authors.

We also want to thank Karger publishers for their idea and their support in producing this book.

*Klaus Rose*
*John N. van den Anker*

...

# The Editors

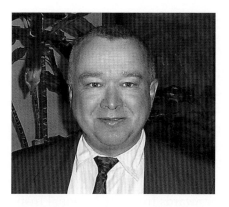 *Dr. Klaus Rose* was born in Heidelberg, Germany. He qualified in medicine in Berlin after initial studies in Romance languages and psychology leading to an MS in psychology. He completed his post-graduate clinical training in General Medicine in Germany and England before joining the pharmaceutical industry in 1991. Since then, he has held various positions in clinical development of progressively increasing responsibility culminating in the position of Head of Paediatrics in Clinical Development and Medical Affairs at Novartis in Basel. In 2005, he joined Roche Medical Science as Global Head of Paediatrics to establish a focus for excellence in paediatric drug development.

He is married with two daughters. His private interests include Mediterranean-style cooking, good wine, gardening, Romance languages, and classical guitar.

He is a frequent speaker on national and international conferences on paediatric drug development including academic conferences, the EFGCP (European Forum for Good Clinical Practice), the DIA (Drug Information Association), the ECPM (European Course of Pharmaceutical Medicines) and others. He also serves as chairman to the EFGCP children's medicines working party.

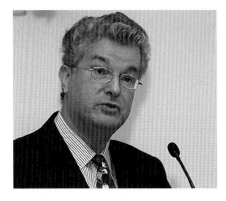

*John N. van den Anker* received his Medical Degree in 1983 from Erasmus University, Rotterdam, The Netherlands, and was a resident in Paediatrics (1984–1988) and a fellow in Neonatal Medicine (1999–2001) at Sophia Children's Hospital in Rotterdam, The Netherlands. After his clinical training he conducted clinical pharmacology studies investigating the impact of renal function development on clinical pharmacokinetics in the neonate that resulted in the successful defence of his PhD in 1995. In 1999, he became Director of Neonatology and Professor of Paediatrics and Neonatology at Erasmus University.

Currently, he is the Director of Pediatric Clinical Pharmacology at the Children's National Medical Center in Washington, D.C., USA and is Professor of Pediatrics, Pharmacology and Physiology at George Washington University School of Medicine and Health Sciences. He is also appointed at the Erasmus Medical Center as a Professor of Pediatrics and Pediatric Clinical Pharmacology. Since 2005, he holds the Evan and Cindy Jones Chair in Pediatric Clinical Pharmacology at the Children's National Medical Center.

He has been granted several major awards from the National Institute of Health (NIH) and leads one of the 13 Pediatric Pharmacology Research Units in the USA.

He has published over 150 peer-reviewed papers in the field of neonatal and paediatric clinical pharmacology and serves on the Editorial Board of several Clinical Pharmacology journals.

His continued commitment and active participation in paediatric clinical pharmacology in Europe has resulted in his election as President of the European Society of Developmental, Perinatal and Paediatric Pharmacology (2006–2008) and he will host the next meeting of this Society in June 4–7, 2008 in Rotterdam, The Netherlands.

Supported in part by grants 1K24RR019729, National Center for Research Resources and 1U10HD45993, National Institute of Child Health and Development, Bethesda, Md., USA

The Editors

······················
# Authors' Short Biographies

*Jörg Breitkreutz*

Prof. Breitkreutz qualified in pharmacy in Münster, Germany. He completed his PhD in Münster at the Institute of Pharmaceutics and Biopharmaceutics in 1996 before joining the pharmaceutical company Thiemann Arzneimittel, Waltrop, Germany, of the Organon/Akzo Nobel group for 2 years. Moving back to university he worked on oral drug formulations for paediatric use finishing his habilitation thesis on this topic in 2004. In 2004 he became a full professor for Pharmaceutical Technology and Biopharmaceutics at the Heinrich Heine University in Düsseldorf, Germany. His main research area is the development of drug formulations and drug delivery devices for paediatrics and geriatrics and for orphan drugs.

*Oscar E. Della Pasqua*

Director in Clinical Pharmacology & Discovery Medicine at GlaxoSmithKline in the United Kingdom and Associate Professor at the Division of Pharmacology at the Leiden/Amsterdam Center for Drug Research in The Netherlands. Following his initial studies in medicine and pharmaceutical sciences, he obtained his PhD degree in Pharmacology at the University of Leiden, The Netherlands. In addition to his extensive experience in early and late clinical development, Dr. Della Pasqua is also a scientific advisor in paediatric drug development and member of the Executive Board of TEDDY, the European network of excellence in medicines for children, under the auspices of the European Union.

*Patricia A. Fowler*

She has worked in the pharmaceutical industry for over 20 years. During this time she has had experience in a research clinic, conducting healthy volunteer studies and also within Clinical Pharmacology involved in the development of Drug Development Plans and Protocols to support products in a number of therapeutic areas. She is currently coordinating support to project teams with queries in their paediatric drug development programmes.

*Sabine Fürst-Recktenwald*

Clinical Research Director in the Clinical & Exploratory Pharmacology Department at sanofi-aventis. She is responsible for the clinical pharmacology part of clinical development plans and pharmacodynamic studies. Additionally, she is chairman of the international clinical development paediatric network within sanofi-aventis.

Prior to this she was European Scientific Director for Diabetes at Aventis EU Medical and Medical Advisor for Diabetology and Metabolism at Aventis Germany. She has broad experience in the management of international paediatric trials.

Dr. Fürst-Recktenwald is trained in medicine at the Universities of Freiburg and Würzburg in Germany and is specialized in paediatrics at the Paediatric Department of the Universities of Würzburg, Heidelberg and Erlangen in Germany. She is a diabetologist according to the German Diabetes Association.

*Marietta M. Henry*

Dr. Henry graduated from medical school at Indiana University in the US after receiving an AB degree in zoology and a Masters degree in pathology, also at Indiana University. She then joined the paediatric program at Indiana University. After 8 years practicing paediatrics in private practice, student health and public health, she returned to the Indiana University Medical Center and completed training for certification in anatomic and clinical pathology and a subspecialty certification in medical microbiology. She worked in clinical pathology in Nebraska at a tertiary care hospital for 11 years and then joined Covance Clinical Laboratory Services, a central laboratory for pharmaceutical clinical trials, where she has been Vice President, Medical Affairs and Global Medical Director for the past 16 years.

*Alastair Kent*

Director of the Genetic Interest Group (GIG) – the UK alliance of charities and support groups for people affected by genetic disorders. GIG's mission is to promote the development of the scientific understanding of genetics and the part that genetic factors play in health and disease, and to see the speedy transfer of this new knowledge into improved services and support for the treatment of currently incurable conditions.

Prior to joining GIG, Alastair worked for a number of voluntary organisations on issues concerning policy, service development and disabled people.

*Pirjo Laitinen-Parkkonen*

Specialist in paediatric anesthesiology, intensive care and pain management. She has focused on paediatric issues in her clinical work and research for more than 10 years. She is now a clinical assessor in the National Agency for Medicines, Finland

*Jane Lamprill*

Jane is an independent Paediatric Research Consultant based near Oxford, UK. Trained at Great Ormond Street Children's Hospital in London, she has 16 years experience as a Paediatric Research Sister (Senior Study Site Coordinator) managing both pharmaceutical, community and academic paediatric clinical trials. Seven of these years were as Paediatric Research Sister at the Royal Brompton & Harefield NHS Trust and Imperial College, London. Her current research with them as co-investigator, is a questionnaire project entitled 'Retrospective investigation into attitudes and experiences of child and parent respiratory clinical trial participants, to inform future best practice'.

She was Paediatric Research Advisor to Origin Pharmaceuticals Ltd (now Constella Group) in 2003 and founded Paediatric Research Consultancy in June 2004. In her consultancy role, Jane collaborates with companies by advising on the Ethics Committee aspects of paediatric trials and gives practical advice on trial protocols and management to help speed up time to market.

Jane provides an ethical, child-centred approach to enable a better trial experience for the children and families which increases recruitment and compliance. She is also a published children's author and writes clear, child friendly information sheets. These have been translated for paediatric trials around the world to facilitate informed consent and assent. Her previous publications can be found at www.janelamp.co.uk.

### Samuel Maldonado

Dr. Maldonado graduated from Medical School at the National University of Honduras, Central America. He then completed his paediatric residency at Henry Ford Hospital in Detroit, Mich., USA followed by a combined fellowship in Pediatric Infectious Diseases at Children's Medical Center in Washington, D.C., USA, and a Regulatory Sciences fellowship at the Food and Drug Administration in Rockville, Md., USA. He served as Medical Officer at the FDA reviewing multiple NDAs and INDs for a total of 8 years. Upon leaving the FDA he joined Boehringer-Ingelheim where he worked in Clinical Virology. From 2000 to 2006 he worked at Johnson & Johnson in Pediatric Drug Development and Global Regulatory Affairs. In April 2006 he joined Wyeth Research as Assistant Vice President and Therapeutic Area Head in Global Regulatory Affairs.

### Dirk Matthys

Dr. Matthys qualified in medicine at the University of Ghent, Belgium, and completed his postgraduate training in paediatrics at the University Hospital, Ghent, followed by a training in paediatric cardiology in Ghent and London. He is chairman of the Department of Paediatrics and secretary of the Ethics Committee of the University Hospital, Ghent.

### David Neubauer

Dr. Neubauer completed his medical studies at Ljubljana University in 1977 and thereafter accomplished his postgraduate study in paediatrics in 1984. He completed his PhD thesis on cardiorespirographic studies in neonates and infants in 1993 and has had further education on neonatal and infantile neurophysiological studies in Lyon and Paris. His other main areas of interest are neonatal neurology and neurodegenerative diseases as well as bioethics in paediatrics, especially ethical problems in handicapped children. At present he is the Head of Child, Adolescent

& Developmental Neurology Department and Professor in Paediatrics at University Medical Center, Children's Hospital, Ljubljana, Slovenia, and since 2005 president of the Ethics working group at CESP/EAP.

### Cor Oosterwijk

Since its foundation in 2004, Cor Oosterwijk (1962) has been Vice President of the European Genetic Alliances' Network (EGAN, www.egaweb.org). EGAN is the European association of patient organisations with a specific interest in genetics, genomics and biomedical research. One of the founders of EGAN is the Dutch Genetic Alliance (VSOP, www.vsop.nl; www.erfelijkheid.nl) of which Oosterwijk is the Executive Director. To serve its 60 member patient organizations that are dealing with genetic, congenital and rare diseases, the VSOP is active in the field of community genetics, genomics and rare diseases, in healthcare policy, in education and public awareness.

Oosterwijk's national positions include member of the Foundation for Preconception Care, member of the scientific advisory board of the Centre for Society and Genomics (CSG), and member of the advisory board of the Paediatric Pharmacotherapy Network and the Medicines for Children Network. Oosterwijk studied Medical Biology at Utrecht University. In earlier positions, he was a Senior Clinical Trial Manager and teacher of Biotechnological Engineering. Cor Oosterwijk is married and father of two sons of which the oldest has Down syndrome.

### Gerard Pons

Prof. Pons graduated MD from the University Xavier Bichat in Paris, France. He trained in Paediatrics during a 4-year residency in Paris and was Assistant Professor in Paediatrics for 3 years. He spent 2 years as Post-Doctoral Research Fellow in Paediatric Clinical Pharmacology in the University of Minnesota (USA). He spent 3 years as Assistant Professor and 4 years as Associate Professor in Paediatric Clinical Pharmacology in the University René Descartes in Paris. He graduated with a PhD in Pharmacology. He has been Professor in Pharmacology since 1991 and Head of the Perinatal and Paediatric Pharmacology Department in the Hospital Saint-Vincent de Paul (University René Descartes) in Paris since 1996. He was General Secretary of the European Society for Developmental Pharmacology from 1994 to 2001. He is a founding member of the European Network for Drug Investigation in Children

(ENDIC). He is a member of the Paediatric Working Party (PEG) of the CHMP at EMEA. His main current research interests are in maturation of drug metabolism and drug development for children with a special emphasis on promoting innovative methodologies in order to circumvent the challenges faced in developing medical products for children.

*Ysbrand Poortman*

A biologist by education and the father of a daughter born with a serious genetic condition.

He founded on the national level an association for neuromuscular disorders (VSN, Baarn) and an alliance of genetic support groups (VSOP, Soestdijk, 1975) of which he was the executive director up till 2002. He co-founded alliances at the European level (European Genetic Alliances' Network, 1991) and at the global level (International Genetic Alliance, 2000).

He also co-founded an international research support organization for neuromuscular disorders (ENMC, Baarn, 1989) and the World Alliance of Organizations for the Prevention and Treatment of Genetic and Congenital Conditions (WAO, New York, 1994).

He co-founded (Brussels, 1994) and chaired (from 2002 up till 2006) the European Platform Patient Organisations, Science and Industry (EPPOSI).

He has served in various advisory boards (e.g. Dutch National Health Council), academic councils and expert committees.

He has authored a large number of publications such as a handbook on neuromuscular diseases, chapters in books, articles, teaching packages, and information material on genetics.

*José Ramet*

Prof. Ramet received his MD and PhD degrees from the Vrije Universiteit, Brussels in Belgium and did his paediatric residency training at the Academic Hospital VUB.

Prof. Ramet is currently Professor at the Universiteit Antwerpen and chairman of the Departments of Paediatrics at the University Hospital of Antwerp (UZA) and the Paola Children's Hospital ZNA, both located in Antwerp.

Prof. Ramet has made diverse contributions in the field of paediatrics publishing over 50 original research articles in peer-reviewed journals. He has worked on many aspects of paediatrics.

His main research interest is in the area of autonomic nervous system control mechanisms, artificial ventilation and vaccination. His research has led to the development of newer and more effective ventilation techniques in children. Future research efforts are directed to new therapeutic strategies in the field of paediatrics.

He is the first president of the European Board of Paediatrics; he is also Secretary-General of CESP (European Confederation of Specialists in Paediatrics/European Academy of Paediatrics), Past-President of the European Society of Paediatric and Neonatal Intensive Care and a member of several scientific societies.

On a national level, he is Vice President of the Belgian Paediatric Society and member of the Founding Committee of the Belgian Paediatric Drug Network (BPDN).

He has served on many international and national committees regarding research and training in paediatrics.

He is a past or present member of the editorial board for several journals and at present member of the Editorial Boards of *Pediatrics* and *Pediatric Critical Care Medicine* and reviewer of several international publications. He has given over 100 presentations at international congresses and meetings.

*Klaus Rose*
Dr. Rose qualified in medicine in Berlin after initial studies in Romance languages and psychology in Heidelberg, Florence and Berlin leading to an MS in psychology. He completed his postgraduate clinical training in General Medicine in Germany and England before joining the pharmaceutical industry in 1991. He has held various positions in clinical development of progressively increasing responsibility. In 2005, he joined Roche Medical Science as Head of Paediatrics.

*Tsveta Schyns*

Dr. Schyns founded the European Network for Research on Alternating Hemiplegia, ENRAH, in the spring of 2003 in Vienna, Austria. She is at present the co-ordinator of the EU-funded project 'ENRAH for SMEs' and Board member of EGAN (European Genetic Alliances Network).

Before that, she pursued an academic career at the Free University of Amsterdam, The Netherlands.

Tsveta Schyns was trained in Molecular Biology at the University of Sofia, Bulgaria. She specialised and conducted her post-graduate studies at the University of Wageningen, The Netherlands, where in 1998 she received her doctor's degree in Genetics.

Tsveta Schyns is married and has two daughters. They currently live in Vienna, Austria.

*Marianne Soergel*

Dr. Soergel studied Medicine in Geneva and Basel, and was trained as a Paediatrician in Heidelberg (Germany). She has worked in patient care and clinical research in Paediatric University Hospitals for 15 years, including 8 years as a consultant in Paediatric Nephrology in Marburg (Germany). She joined Clinical Research and Development at Novartis in 2001, and has been an active member of the Novartis Paediatric Advisory Group since 2002. She has two school-aged children.

*Despina Solomonidou*

Head of Global Project Coordination in Technical Research & Development at Novartis Pharma AG in Basel, Switzerland. A pharmaceutical scientist by training, Dr. Solomonidou holds a PhD in Pharmaceutical Technology. With her 10 years of industrial experience in drug product design and development, she has became well established as senior expert for paediatric drug product development with advanced knowledge of patient needs and business requirements. In partnership with other industry and academic experts, she elaborated a reflection paper on paediatric formulations on behalf of the Paediatric Expert Group of CHMP.

*Philippe Steenhout*

Dr. Steenhout obtained his diploma of medicine at the Free University of Brussels (ULB) in 1982. He practiced general medicine for 2 years, and then continued his postgraduate clinical training, obtaining a license in Paediatrics in 1989. After having worked as a clinician with research and teaching responsibilities in Belgium, he joined the Nestlé Headquarters in Switzerland in 1993 as medical advisor for the infant nutrition business. Since 2005 he is head of the Department of Medical and Clinical Development within Nestlé Nutrition.

*Hans Stötter*

Dr. Stötter has a degree in internal medicine with subspecialization in haematology and oncology, and a diploma in pharmaceutical medicine. After several years in research in Immunology and Oncology, he worked for Ciba in Basel before joining the former IKS (now Swissmedic), the Swiss agency for therapeutic products as clinical reviewer. Since 8/2004 he is head of the paediatric working group of Swissmedic.

*Catherine Tuleu*

Dr. Tuleu is a UK-qualified French pharmacist (Université Paris V and XI). After a post-doctoral fellowship and a first lecturing appointment in the UK, she joined the Centre for Paediatric Pharmacy Research in 2003 at the School of Pharmacy, University of London as Paediatric Drug Delivery Lecturer. She is now Deputy Director of the centre. Closely with specialised hospitals, one aspect of Catherine's work is to ensure that medicines for children are effective, safe and of quality and to stimulate innovative research in paediatric formulation. With a background in Pharmaceutical Technology and Biopharmaceutics, the generic theme of her research is gastrointestinal drug delivery with emphasis on colonic targeting where she developed expertise ranging from in vitro, animal and clinical evaluation (gamma-scintigraphy).

*John N. van den Anker*

Professor van den Anker received his medical degree in 1983 from Erasmus University, Rotterdam, the Netherlands, and was a resident in Paediatrics (1984–1988) and a fellow in Neonatal Medicine (1999–2001) at Sophia Children's Hospital in Rotterdam, the Netherlands. After his clinical training he conducted clinical pharmacology studies in the neonate that resulted in the successful defence of his PhD in 1995. In 1999, he became Director of Neonatology and Professor of Paediatrics and Neonatology at Erasmus University.

Currently, he is the Director of Pediatric Clinical Pharmacology at the Children's National Medical Center in Washington, D.C., USA and is Professor of Pediatrics, Pharmacology and Physiology at George Washington University School of Medicine and Health Sciences. Since 2005, he holds the Evan and Cindy Jones Chair in Pediatric Clinical Pharmacology at the Children's National Medical Center.

He has been granted several major awards from the National Institute of Health (NIH) and has published over 150 peer-reviewed papers in the field of neonatal and paediatric clinical pharmacology.

He serves currently as President of the European Society of Developmental, Perinatal and Paediatric Pharmacology.

### Ekhard Ziegler

Dr. Ziegler attended medical school and received his paediatric training at the University of Innsbruck. He trained in paediatric nutrition with Samuel Fomon and has been on the faculty of the Department of Pediatrics, University of Iowa, since 1973. His area of interest and expertise is the nutrition of infants, both preterm and fullterm. His current research interest focuses on the breastfed infant, where he is exploring ways to prevent iron and vitamin D deficiency.

### Lothar-Bernd Zimmerhackl

Professor Zimmerhackl qualified in medicine, mathematics, physics and chemistry in Berlin and Heidelberg, Germany. He finished his thesis in physiology and did his postdoctoral training in nephrology and paediatrics in Stanford (USA), Heidelberg, Marburg and Freiburg (Germany). He has specialized training in paediatric nephrology, neonatology and paediatric intensive care.

Since 2002 he is chairman of the Department for Pediatric I at the Medical University Innsbruck (Austria).

# Authors' Addresses

**Prof. Dr. Jörg Breitkreutz**
Professor for Pharmaceutical Technology
Heinrich Heine University Düsseldorf
Institute of Pharmaceutics and Biopharmaceutics
Universitätsstrasse 1
DE–40225 Düsseldorf (Germany)
Tel. +49 211 811 0678, Fax +49 211 811 4251
E-Mail joerg.breitkreutz@uni-duesseldorf.de

**Dr. Oscar E. Della Pasqua**
Clinical Pharmacology & Discovery Medicine
GlaxoSmithKline
Greenford Road
Greenford UB6 0HE (UK)
Tel. +44 20 8966 2404, Fax +44 20 8966 2123
E-Mail odp72514@gsk.com

**Sabine Fürst-Recktenwald, MD**
Clinical Research Director
Clinical and Exploratory Pharmacology
Sanofi-Aventis Deutschland GmbH
Industriepark Höchst, Building H 831
DE–65926 Frankfurt am Main (Germany)
Tel. +49 69 305 28053, Fax +49 69 305 17230
E-Mail Sabine.Fuerst-Recktenwald@sanofi-aventis.com

**Marietta M. Henry, MD**
Vice President, Medical Affairs and Global Laboratory Medical Director
Covance Central Laboratory Services
8211 SciCor Drive
Indianapolis, IN 46214 (USA)
Tel. +1 317 273 7934, Fax +1 317 273 7990
E-Mail Marietta.Henry@Covance.com

**Alastair Kent**
Director
Genetic Interest Group
4D Leroy House
436 Essex Road
London N1 3QP (UK)
Tel. +44 20 7704 3141, Fax +44 20 7359 1447
E-Mail alastair@gig.org.uk
www.gig.org.uk

**Pirjo Laitinen-Parkkonen, MD, PhD**
National Agency for Medicines
Mannerheimintie 103b
FI–00301 Helsinki (Finland)
Tel. +358 9 473 34 411
E-Mail Pirjo.Laitinen-Parkkonen@nam.fi

**Jane Lamprill**
Paediatric Research Consultant
Paediatric Research Consultancy
E-Mail prc@janelamp.co.uk
www.janelamp.co.uk

**Samuel D. Maldonado, MD, MPH**
PhRMA Chair, Pediatric Committee and Assistant Vice President
Global Regulatory Affairs
Therapeutic Area Head
Women's Health
Wyeth Research
500 Arcola Road
Collegeville, PA 19426 (USA)
Tel. +1 484 865 2667, Fax +1 484 865 4312
E-Mail maldons@wyeth.com

**Dirk Matthys**
Department of Pediatrics
Ghent University
De Pintelaan 185
BE–9000 Ghent (Belgium)
Tel. +32 9 240 35 84, Fax +32 9 240 38 75
E-Mail dirk.matthys@ugent.be

**Dr. David Neubauer**
University Children's Hospital Ljubljana
Department of Child, Adolescent and Developmental Neurology
Vrazov trg 1
SI-1525 Ljubljana (Slovenia)
Tel. +386 1 522 9273, Fax +386 1 522 9357
E-Mail david.neubauer@mf.uni-lj.si
www.kclj.si/pednevro

**Dr. Cor Oosterwijk**
Vice-president EGAN, Director VSOP
Vredehofstraat 31
NL–3761 HA Soestdijk (The Netherlands)
Tel. +31 35 603 4040, Fax +31 35 602 7440
E-Mail c.oosterwijk@vsop.nl
www.egaweb.org, www.vsop.nl

**Gerard Pons, MD, PhD**
Pharmacologist, Paediatrician
Professor of Clinical Pharmacology
University René Descartes
Head Clinical Pharmacology
Cochin – Saint Vincent de Paul Hospital
82, Avenue Denfert-Rochereau
FR–75674 Paris Cedex 14 (France)
Tel. +33 1 4048 8219, Fax +33 1 4048 8328
E-Mail gerard.pons@svp.ap-hop-paris.fr

**Ysbrand Poortman**
Secretary General International Genetic Alliance of
parent and patient organisations (IGA)
Vice President World Alliance of Organizations for Prevention
and Treatment of Genetic and Congenital Conditions (WAO)
Helios 130, Gerstkamp
NL–2592 CV The Hague (The Netherlands)
Tel. +31 35 683 1920, Fax +31 35 602 7440
E-Mail y.poortman@vsop.nl

**Prof. José Ramet**
Chairman Department of Pediatrics
University Hospital of Antwerp (UZA)
Wilrijkstraat 10
BE–2650 Edegem (Belgium)
Tel. +32 3 821 4015, Fax +32 3 821 4300
E-Mail jose.ramet@uza.be

and

ZNA Queen Paola Children Hospital
Lindendreef
BE–2020 Antwerp (Belgium)
Tel. +32 3 280 2131, Fax +32 3 280 2132
E-Mail jose.ramet@zna.be

**Klaus Rose, MD, MS**
Head Pediatrics
F. Hoffmann-La Roche Ltd.
Pharmaceuticals Division, PDM5
CH–4070 Basel (Switzerland)
E-Mail klaus.rose@roche.com

**Dr. Tsveta Schyns**
ENRAH Association
Tivoligasse 70/10
AT–1120 Vienna (Austria)
Tel./Fax +43 1 920 0075, Mobile +43 699 1920 0192
E-Mail ts@enrah.net
www.enrah.net

**Marianne Soergel, MD**
WSJ 157 – 3.15
Novartis Pharma AG
CH–4002 Basel (Switzerland)
Tel. +41 61 324 23 90, Fax +41 61 324 49 39
E-Mail marianne.soergel@novartis.com

**Dr. Despina Solomonidou**
Head of Global Technical R&D Project Coordination
Novartis Pharma AG
Pharma Development
Forum 3.1.100
Postfach
CH–4002 Basel (Switzerland)
E-Mail despina.solomonidou@novartis.com

**Philippe Steenhout, PhD, MD**
Head Medical & Clinical Development
Nestlé Nutrition
Nestec Ltd.
REL 321-07
Av. Reller 22
CH–1800 Vevey (Switzerland)
E-Mail philippe.steenhout@nestle.com

**Hans Stötter, MD**
Swissmedic
Hallerstr. 7
CH–3100 Bern (Switzerland)
Tel. +41 31 322 03 39
E-Mail Hans.Stoetter@swissmedic.ch

**Dr. Catherine Tuleu**
Lecturer in Pharmaceutics
Deputy Director Centre for Paediatric Pharmacy Research
The School of Pharmacy
University of London
29–39 Brunswick Square
London WC1N 1AX (UK)
Tel. +44 207 753 5857, Fax +44 207 753 5942
E-Mail catherine.tuleu@pharmacy.ac.uk

**John N. van den Anker, MD, PhD**
Center for Clinical Research and Experimental Therapeutics
Children's Research Institute
Children's National Medical Center
111 Michigan Avenue, NW
Washington, DC 20010 (USA)
E-Mail jvandena@cnmc.org

and

Department of Pediatrics
Erasmus MC – Sophia Children's Hospital
Dr. Molewaterplein 60
NL–3015 GJ Rotterdam (The Netherlands)

**Prof. Ekhard Ziegler**
Department of Pediatrics
University of Iowa
200 Hawkins Drive
Iowa City, IA 52242-1083 (USA)
Tel. +1 319 356 1831, Fax +1 319 356 8669
E-Mail ekhard-ziegler@uiowa.edu

**Prof. Lothar-Bernd Zimmerhackl**
Department of Pediatrics I
Medical University Innsbruck
Anichstraße 35
AT–6020 Innsbruck (Austria)
Tel. +43 512 504 23501, Fax +43 512 504 25450
E-Mail lothar-bernd.zimmerhackl@uki.at

Rose K, van den Anker JN (eds): Guide to Paediatric Clinical Research.
Basel, Karger, 2007, pp 1–4

........................

# Europe's Path towards Better Medicines for Children

*José Ramet*[a]    *Klaus Rose*[b]

[a]University of Antwerp, Universitair Ziekenhuis Antwerpen UZA and ZNA, Paola Children's Hospital, Antwerp, Belgium;
[b]Pediatrics, F. Hoffmann-La Roche Ltd., Pharmaceuticals Division, Basel, Switzerland

The goal of modern medicine is to be able to treat conditions for which there would have been absolutely no hope of recovery decades and centuries ago. The armamentarium of today includes modern diagnostic tools, drugs, operation techniques, and devices of all sorts, to name but a few. The physician will always play the key role in deciding and delivering the most appropriate treatment but recently many steps in the therapeutic approach and in the physician-patient relationship have evolved and are still developing, making the whole process more and more complex. Since the beginning of the 1960s government action has forced pharmaceutical companies in Europe to provide scientific evidence on efficacy and safety of all new drugs. This has led to standards of clinical testing within the Good Clinical Practice (GCP) framework that are now recognized worldwide and are still evolving as a global process (ICH E 6 – GCP: www.ich.org/LOB/media/MEDIA482.pdf). Drug development has become a complex interdisciplinary and global process driven by individual competitive pharmaceutical companies. The registration of modern drugs still remains in the hands of national authorities. A worldwide framework of standardized preclinical, clinical, and technical development and submission procedures has evolved within the International Conference on Harmonisation of Technical Requirements for Registration of Pharmaceuticals for Human Use which is now binding for all major national health authorities (ICH – International Conference on Harmonisation: www.ich.org).

Still, treating patients within the framework of clinical trials relies on the infrastructure and logistics of the particular pharmaceutical company that drives drug development.

Children have, however, not profited as much as adults from the therapeutic benefits that this dynamic process increasingly offers. The reasons for this are complex and involve many aspects of society and people's thoughts and feelings. Today nobody would challenge that it was courageous and positive when a new treatment regimen of cytotoxic drugs was administered to children with acute lymphatic leukemia from the 1970s on. However, in those days the paediatric oncologists were accused of using the children as 'guinea pigs'. It is now broadly accepted that new treatment opportunities should be available to our children once their efficacy and safety has been proven. Public opinion is nevertheless not always aware that these regimens require the treatment of children within clinical trials. Although every effort has been undertaken to minimize the risks and adverse events in paediatric clinical trials, it is impossible to exclude every imaginable risk with a 100% safety margin. A careful balance between risk and potential gain in therapeutic benefit or at least therapeutic knowledge will always be part of clinical testing, in children as well as in adults.

A new reflection supports the inclusion of children into the general drug development process since all medicines used in children should be systematically tested in the various age groups. This thinking was behind the paediatric legislations introduced in the USA since the 1990s. It contributed to a better knowledge of the metabolism and physiological processes in infants and children, and a growing understanding of the rights children have as part of our society. In the USA, pragmatic thinking has found a way to for funding the additional investments required for paediatric research.

Today Europe is being perceived more and more as a regional entity comparable to the USA and Japan in its strength and importance.

To what degree is this true for research in paediatrics, in the field of paediatric clinical trials, or in the world of therapeutic innovations for newborns, infants and children? In contrast to several decades ago, today a medical doctor trained in any country belonging to the European Union can work in any other EU country without having to pass additional examinations that require years of preparation. In the EMEA (European Agency for the Evaluation of Medicinal Products), Europe now has a central drug evaluation agency. This organization is, however, not completely comparable with the FDA, as it is a coordinating institution on top of the existing national drug registration authorities. In certain countries, the national paediatric organisations play still bigger roles than the European umbrella organisation, the European Academy of Paediatrics (EAP), that has evolved from its predecessor the CESP (Confederation of European Specialists in Paediatrics). In their professional activities, the majority of European paediatricians still see themselves as nationals of their respective countries, although the weight of European institutions is now gradually increasing. Parallel to the introduction in the USA of the FDA Modernization Act (FDAMA) in 1997 and the Pediatric Rule in 1998, a debate on better medicines for children also started in Europe. Considerable time was taken before reaching a stage that has practical consequences; this might be symptomatic for Europe. Several national governments, initially specifically in France, have put this topic very high on their agendas. Conversely, individual European countries, as big as France or as small as Belgium, no longer have the full potential to seriously influence decisions on drug development in globally acting companies. The idea to offer pharmaceutical companies financial incentives for additional paediatric research on top of mandatory paediatric requirements was adapted from the positive US experience on this issue. This progressed to a real European idea, no longer triggered by one or several national governments, but directly promoted by the European Commission in constructive association with the EMEA – after an initial declaration of the EU Health Council. The EU paediatric regulation also reflects the long path Europe will have to take to get one voice and be able to set directions worldwide. Several national paediatric research networks are being developed, the UK MCRN (http://mcrn.org.uk/) and the German PaedNet (www.paed-net.org/) being the most advanced. At least two initiatives are trying to build up a truly European Paediatric Research Network – MediChildren (www.medichildren.net/) and TEDDY (www.teddyoung.org). National networks are often still underdeveloped and will have to adapt to new conditions where the financial input of state funds will no longer be guaranteed.

The pharmaceutical market in Europe is far from uniform. Each country has one or several competing health insurance and reimbursement systems; medical care is partially private and frequently state owned. The rewards for paediatric research are assigned to the member states with their respective different markets – a complex challenge for every company that wants to deal with these incentives. At least the duration of the planned protection against generic competition will have the same time frame in every single European country. All paediatric investigations plans (PIPs) will be handled centrally by the EMEA Paediatric Committee (PC).

The introduction of the EU paediatric regulation is a starting point: the real work is yet to come. European paediatricians, regulators and pharmaceutical companies have lobbied for this legislation. However, several questions remain unanswered: To what degree will the EMEA Paediatric Committee (PC) award additional paediatric research if basic data are already available through the FDA-triggered research programs? Will the EMEA accept research on rare diseases, as done by the FDA that granted paediatric exclusivity to Tamoxifen for the research in McCune-Albright syndrome? How will the implementation guidelines for the PUMA program be introduced? Will the EMEA PC spend considerable time screening existing paediatric trials on the available databases in order to prevent unnecessary trials? Or will this be done by the Ethical Committees? How will the Ethical Committees coordinate their function across the European member countries? How many years will it still take until one vote of a European Ethical Committee is sufficient for a paediatric clinical trial performed in several European countries?

Although child health in Europe has never been as good as it is today, there is still plenty of room for improvement. Europe represents a huge platform of knowledge, science, wealth, and education. In international, global competition Europe lags behind in its abilities to make full use of its capacities. Although it may be difficult to resolve the problems encountered on a day-to-day basis, in the end it will be the job of European researchers to move this region forward, both in the interests of our citizens and those of our children.

Rose K, van den Anker JN (eds): Guide to Paediatric Clinical Research.
Basel, Karger, 2007, pp 5–12

··········

# The European Academy of Paediatrics (EAP/CESP) and Its Demand for More Clinical Research

*José Ramet*[a]   *John N. van den Anker*[b]

[a]University of Antwerp, Universitair Ziekenhuis Antwerpen UZA and ZNA, Paola Children's Hospital, Antwerp, Belgium;
[b]Division of Pediatric Clinical Pharmacology, Children's National Medical Center, and Departments of Pediatrics, Pharmacology and Physiology, George Washington University School of Medicine and Health Sciences, Washington, D.C., USA, and Department of Pediatrics, Erasmus MC – Sophia Children's Hospital, Rotterdam, The Netherlands

## Introduction

There are more than 100 million children in the 25 countries of the recently enlarged European Union (EU). The majority of parents of these children are not aware that medicines are often not tested, labelled, or approved for the indications for which they are prescribed by paediatricians. Likewise, most policymakers in Europe assume that the same standards of quality, safety and efficacy are applied to children's as to adult medicines.

In their daily working life, physicians and especially paediatricians are often confronted with a dilemma when they have to decide on the treatment of a child: off-label use of a drug or no use?

When a drug is approved by regulatory authorities, indications and dosages are part of the information leaflet. It is only in these situations that the risk-benefit ratio has been reviewed and accepted by the regulatory authorities. In any other circumstances, the drug is used outside the limits of its label, with the result that neither the pharmaceutical com-

pany nor the authorities have any legal or ethical responsibility for unexpected adverse events. Different dosages, use outside the labelled indications, modifications of the pharmaceutical form (breaking up tablets to prepare capsules with smaller amounts of the drug or making
solutions for children are considered 'special formulations') or modifications related to the route of administration (i.v. solutions for oral or in-
trathecal use) are all examples of unapproved uses and are part of the
daily routine [1].

The European Commission, the European Parliament and the
Council approved the European legislation on paediatric medicines.
This will help provide better medicines for Europe's children and increase paediatric research in Europe, especially clinical trials. Over the
next few months all stakeholders need to get ready for action.


## The FDA Model?

There have been a variety of reasons why more extensive paediatric
testing has not been conducted despite its importance for public health.
The drug industry did not have incentives to develop drugs for paediatric use because of the comparatively small size of the paediatric market
for most products. The lack of adequate legal protection from liability
problems that might occur during paediatric trials is an additional reason for the scarcity of paediatric studies.

Designing and completing paediatric research trials for medicines
can also present scientific, ethical, and logistical challenges such as recruiting sufficient study participants and obtaining consent from parents or guardians or developing appropriate formulations of a drug that
can be administered to younger patients. All these obstacles resulted in
the fact that, before 1997, regulatory efforts to address the lack of paediatric studies and insufficient labelling information had been largely unsuccessful [2].

The FDA therefore developed incentives for pharmaceutical companies to perform pharmaceutical research. This has resulted in the
achievement of this goal of paediatric research and as a consequence labelling for many products have been achieved [3].

In summarising their experience with the legislation to Congress,
the FDA called it the most successful instrument ever developed [4]. The

FDA now has the clear authority to require paediatric studies to ensure that drugs are safe and effective for children [5].

For the last 7 years Europe has watched developments in the United States and has taken halting steps to address the paediatric problem in Europe. No specific legislation encouraging pharmaceutical paediatric research exists and this results in a lack of research today in the EU.

In 2002, the European Commission launched a consultation document on Better Medicines for Children and proposed regulatory actions regarding paediatric medicinal products [6].

The intention of this proposal was to provide a legislative framework that would facilitate an improved understanding of safety and efficacy information on medicinal products used in child health.

While dozens of initiatives have supported the paediatric infrastructure in the United States, insufficient paediatric clinical work has been done in Europe. This has contributed to the declining competitiveness of European research and, no doubt, to the steady brain drain of researchers from Europe. Recent data of the European Commission show that despite higher levels of university graduates than in the United States, far fewer researchers find employment in Research and Development in Europe [7].

Several initiatives exist today allowing us to collect information related to the use of medicines in children. A guide with advice on children's medicines is available from the British Medical Association [8].

Pharmacists have done remarkable research to improve the dispensing of children's medicines via extemporaneous formulations. Nevertheless, children and paediatricians need the high level of quality available for licensed medicines [9].

The objectives of the new European regulation are on the one hand to increase the development and authorization of medicines for use in children while ensuring that children's medicines are subject to high quality research, and on the other, there are also safeguards to ensure that children are not subjected to unnecessary clinical trials. At this moment this legislation has to be effectively implemented and applied as soon as possible: paediatricians need paediatric research in Europe [10].

Although this remarkable piece of new legislation is an enormous step forward for the protection of children's health in Europe, it requires a lot of work from the different stakeholders. That is why paediatricians and paediatric organizations, the pharmaceutical industry, the European Parliament, the governments and the EMEA need to prepare its implementation as a prerequisite for success.

As the legislation will result in a growing need for clinical trials, the time to prepare its successful implementation is now.

Several European actors have a crucial role to play in the successful implementation of the new European legislation.

## The Stakeholders and Actors

### EMEA

EMEA has the important role of being the coordinator of the paediatric project. The Paediatric Expert Group at the EMEA defines the public health strategy and priorities, sets the timelines and helps develop the research priorities.

They also need to define clearly how paediatric investigation plans have to be written and submitted and how the study results will be assessed. This is a clear mission behind the legislation and a clear guidance from EMEA is necessary in the coming months.

### Pharmaceutical Industry

The new role for the pharmaceutical industry is to develop clinical programs for the evaluation of medicines in children. They will have to submit paediatric plans answering to the medical needs of the children resulting in improvement of knowledge about the activity of the medicines in children, the adequate dose and dosing schemes related to the age or weight of the child and the risk of adverse drug reactions. There are elements that argue that efforts to improve the quality of pharmacotherapy in children should not exclude widely marketed and firmly established drugs.

### The Ethical Framework

Research is only justified when ethical standards are observed to a high extent. The main ethical principle of all paediatric activities is the demand to do everything in the 'best interests of children'. As a consequence there is not only an ethical demand to be fully aware of the effects of medicinal measures in a general framework, but also a demand to carefully protect the individual child involved in research. Concerning research on medicines the ICH stated that the ethical imperative to obtain knowledge of biomedical data and the effects of medicinal products in paediatric patients has to be balanced against the ethical imperative to protect and respect his or her integrity and personal dignity.

A common ethical framework and operational guidelines for Good Clinical Practice in paediatric research has to correspond as close as possible with the 'best interests of children' and to take into account the continuous increase of ethical questions in our multicultural and pluralistic European societies with different standards of value. The European Academy for Paediatrics/CESP that includes paediatric delegates and specialists of all EU countries approved several documents that have been worked out by its EAP/CESP Ethics Working Group [11–13].

### The European Academy of Paediatrics EAP/CESP and Member States

Paediatricians are the intermediaries between any regulation or research plan and the child. Any paediatric investigation plan will be assessed taking into account the therapeutic benefits and needs for children as laid down by the overall child health strategy put forward by EMEA. Hence, paediatric research centres from all over Europe need to set up partnerships and networks to optimize the undertaking and outcome of the clinical work.

The Member States need to organize the input from the paediatric community for the identification of health priorities in a structured and well-organized manner. In addition, Member States should support the activities related to the paediatric research. On the one side, this support can be structural (how to facilitate networking between paediatricians) and on the other governments need to consider adequate financial support in order to reward the increasing role and responsibility of the paediatricians.

There are opportunities for National governments and EMEA to collaborate through established and developing networks such as the European Academy for Paediatrics (EAP/CESP).

The role of the European Academy for Paediatrics can be to support the Paediatric Expert Group at the EMEA by proposing experienced paediatric experts in the different fields of childhood disease who are able to provide input during the evaluation of the paediatric investigational plans, help define the health priorities that need to be addressed and advise on any other issue related to the implementation of the paediatric regulation or ethical issues.

## Discussion

The objectives of the European legislation on Medicines for children are to improve the health of the children of Europe by increasing high-quality research into medicines for them and to promote the development and authorisation of such medicines.

The design of the new legislation is well tested and reflected in the paediatric rules of the FDA but also in existing European legislation such as the Orphan Drug Regulation [14] and the Supplementary Protection Regulation.

A key reason to support the implementation of this proposal is to improve the information on medicines designed for children, at the same time avoiding unnecessary studies in children and not delaying the authorisation of medicines for adults. Requirements at the time of applications for new medicines are data in children (as agreed by a paediatric committee) or a waiver from the requirement or deferral of the timing of the studies. It will be of utmost importance to keep a very careful eye on the goal of this legislation, which is to foster paediatric pharmaceutical research in order to make better medicines for children available.

The new legislation will require a lot of work from the relevant stakeholders: the pharmaceutical industry, the EMEA, the Member States, paediatricians and the paediatric European organizations.

The role for the pharmaceutical industry is to bring forward satisfactory investigation plans. They have to submit strong plans answering to the medical needs of the children.

As the legislation will result in a growing need for clinical trials, the time to prepare is now. EMEA has the important role of being the coordinator of the paediatric project. EMEA defines the public health strategy and priorities, sets the timelines and helps develop the priorities. The Member States and the paediatric community need to prepare their input in a structured and well-organized manner. Paediatricians are the intermediary between any regulation or research plan and the child. The paediatric investigation plans need to be assessed taking into account the overall child health strategy put forward by EMEA.

Paediatric research centres from all over Europe need to set up partnerships and networks so as to optimize the outcome of the clinical work. Member States should support these activities. This support can be structural – how to facilitate networking between paediatricians – but governments also need to consider financial support in order to reward the increasing role and responsibility of the paediatricians.

There are opportunities for governments and the EMEA to collaborate through established and developing networks such as the European Academy for Paediatrics. The role of the Academy can be to coordinate the efforts of experts in the different fields of childhood disease regarding their input in the evaluation of the paediatric plans, definition of the priorities that need to be addressed, and any other problem related to the paediatric regulation.

Only if all stakeholders work closely together will the legislation provide its optimal results: better health for children. We now have a unique chance to make an important contribution to the organization and support of paediatric research in the EU. All involved partners need to take their responsibility to make this project a success story.

## References

1   Boos J: Editorial. Off label use – label of use? Ann Oncol 2003;14:1–5.
2   Thompson TG, McLellan MG: News Release, 2003. http://www.hhs.gov/news/press/2003pres/20030724.html
3   US Food and Drug Administration: Center for Drug Evaluation and Research. Paediatric Exclusivity Labelling Changes as of August 22, 2003. http://www.fda.gov/cder/pediatric/labelchange.htm
4   The Pediatric Exclusivity Provision: Status Report to Congress –Department of Health and Human. January Services – US Food and Drug Administration, 2001. http://www.fda.gov/cder/pediatric/reportcong01.pdf
5   US Food and Drug Administration: Department of Health and Human Services. FDA Statement. Statement of the FDA Commissioner Mark B. McClellan, MD, PhD, on the signing of the Pediatric Research Equity Act of December 3, 2003. http://www.fda.gov/bbs/topics/NEWS/2003/NEW00989.html
6   European Commission: Pharmaceuticals: regulatory framework and market authorizations. Better medicines for children – proposed regulatory action on paediatric medicinal products. 2002. http://pharmacos.eudra.org/F2/pharmacos/docs/Doc2002/feb/cd_pediatrics_en.pdf

7   European Commission: Directorate-General for Research. Towards a European Research Area Science, Technology and Innovation. Key Figures 2003–2004. 2003, pp 43–44.

8   BNF for Children. bnf.org/bnf/extra/current/noframes/450034.htm

9   Nunn AJ: Making medicines that children can take. Arch Dis Child 2003;88:369–371.

10  Ramet J: What the paediatricians need – the launch of paediatric research in Europe. Eur J Pediatr 2005;164:263–265.

11  Sauer PJJ, members of the Ethics Working Group of CESP: Research in children. Report on behalf of the Ethics Working Group of CESP. Eur J Pediatr 2002;161:1–5.

12  Kurz R: Putting the child first: research as a part of paediatric care. The Joseph Hoet Lecture on Ethics in Paediatric Research. Int J Pharm Med 2002;16:11–13.

13  Kurz R, Gill D, Mjönes, Ethics Working Group of the Confederation of European Specialists in Paediatrics: Ethical issues in the daily medical care of children. Eur J Pediatr 2006;165:83–86.

14  Regulation (EC) No 141/2000 of the European Parliament and of the Council of 16 December 1999 on Orphan Medicinal Products: Official Journal of the European Communities L18, 2000, pp 1–5.

Rose K, van den Anker JN (eds): Guide to Paediatric Clinical Research.
Basel, Karger, 2007, pp 13–24

..........................

# Paediatric Medicines: A View from Patient Organisations

*Alastair Kent*[a]   *Cor Oosterwijk*[b]   *Tsveta Schyns*[d]
*Ysbrand Poortman*[c]

[a]Genetic Interest Group, London, UK; [b]Soestdijk, and [c]Baarn,
The Netherlands; [d]ENRAH Association, Vienna, Austria

## Introduction

For any parents experiencing the arrival of a newborn baby the first question that is asked is 'Is my baby all right?' Fortunately, for most couples, the answer to this question is 'yes', but sadly for some, they cannot be reassured because their baby has a chronic health problem that will potentially limit the quality and possibly the length of life their child can expect.

Even for the parents of a healthy baby the future may be uncertain, as their child will have to face threats to his or her health ranging from the normal diseases of childhood (which are usually relatively mild but which can sometimes be very severe or even fatal) to potentially fatal attacks of meningitis and other violent infectious diseases.

Fortunately, thanks to advances over the last fifty years or so many diseases which were formerly untreatable have become curable as a result of the development of antibiotics and other medicines or preventable by vaccination and other measures to reduce their threat. However, it is still the case today that the vast majority of childhood diseases remain untreatable and the doctor only has recourse to palliation of some of the symptoms when offering care and support to the affected child and his or her family. Many, if not most of these intractable conditions are rare. They usually have a genetic cause, or at least a substantial genetic component, and for the vast majority there is currently little or nothing that can be done to alter their natural course, or change the prognosis for the affected child. Paradoxically, despite the fact that individually these diseases may be rare, because there are many thousands of different conditions (estimates vary, but at least 6,000–8,000 have been described) rare diseases are not uncommon [Online Mendelian Inheritance in Man (OMIM), www.ncbi.nlm.nih.gov], and every doctor will meet some of these during the course of his or her professional life. Some childhood diseases are of course common and for these the need for effective, safe therapies is just as great.

## Research Involving Children

For children affected by currently untreatable disorders hope for the future rests on the undertaking of high quality biomedical research, and the speedy application of the outputs from that research in the form of safe effective medical products – whether drugs, cell or tissue therapies or other forms of innovative intervention targeted at their unmet medical needs.

Using children in research is a sensitive and a contentious issue. The younger the child the more sensitive the issue becomes, because of their inherent vulnerability and their inability to withhold consent to participation. Understandably, there is a fear that parents, desperate for a cure for their sick child, will be pressured into consenting to research that is neither in the interests of their child, nor of others yet to come who have the same condition. Because of this very natural reticence (and for economic reasons too) research into novel medicines for childhood onset diseases has been limited. For the same reasons, medicines developed for diseases of adulthood which start in childhood have often not been properly tested on children prior to being given a Marketing Authorisation by the European Medicines Agency or National Competent Authorities. This leaves doctors in the unenviable position of having to rely on their expertise when deciding appropriate dosages for their paediatric patients, resulting in ineffective treatment. More importantly it leaves already sick children vulnerable to unexpected adverse events occurring due to difference in their ability to metabolise drugs as they grow and develop.

Properly conducted ethically sound research is essential if children with serious health problems are to be able to hope for novel medicines that will alleviate, prevent or cure their condition. Indeed, it is arguable that not to do such research when you have the opportunity to do so is unethical, because it leaves sick children experiencing the impact of diseases which might have become curable, but which, without research, will remain untreatable.

Indeed for many of the rare genetic diseases of childhood there is no option but to do research on children because sadly they do not live long enough to reach adulthood.

The need for high-quality research into medicines for childhood diseases is immense. The opportunity to do this research, in a properly regulated, ethical manner that prospects the interests of the child and safeguards against exploitation is growing. This is a result of the coming together of a number of circumstances which are detailed below.

### Increased Awareness of Rare Childhood Diseases

Largely as a result of recent advances in genetics it has become increasingly possible to provide a definitive diagnosis for growing numbers of rare childhood diseases. This, coupled with the greater understanding of the importance of early, accurate diagnosis for parents and for their children amongst medical professionals has created a climate within which rare diseases are more likely to be visible – and more likely to be on the doctor's 'radar' as something to be looked out for than was the case in the past.

With the advent of diagnosis comes the possibility for patients to come together into self help groups, and (eventually) to develop pressure to promote and conduct research. Even prior to the development of new medicines, accurate diagnosis, coupled with developments in IT (Information Technology) make it possible for patients and their doctors to access up to date information on the 'state of the art' in their disease, for registers to be created and expert centres established able to see a 'critical mass' of patients sufficient to generate knowledge and understanding that can become available to the wider patient and professional community.

There needs to be a systematic effort to raise awareness of parents and the public at large about the importance of paediatric research on how clinical trials in children are carried out. If the first contact a parent has with a clinical trial is the Patient Information Sheet, a valuable opportunity to raise awareness has been lost, and unfortunate pre-conceptions about what is involved may have become fixed and difficult to shift.

Patient organisations and doctors both represent trusted sources of information for the public. Patient organisations in particular are keen to disseminate relevant information to their members (and wider afield too if resourced to do so). Given the opportunity they provide a balanced view of the impact of paediatric research, helping to generate understanding amongst the public and facilitating the recruitment and retention of children to clinical trials and other types of research project.

Sustained engagement rests upon ongoing trust:
- that the doctor will apply current scientific understanding wisely,
- that the pharmaceutical industry will give paediatric R&D a sufficiently high priority,
- that there will be incentives to produce novel therapies for rare conditions where market forces alone will not provide sufficient prospects for a return on investment,
- that governments and the European Institutions will develop a proportionate and appropriate regulatory regime and implement it sensitively and in ways that encourage the production of safe effective therapies for children quickly.


**Keeping up to Date**

It used to be said that you could tell when doctors first qualified by the medicines they prescribed. While this may have been a cruel caricature, it did reflect a serious difficulty in keeping up to date – especially with regard to rare conditions where expertise might be located in disparate centres across the globe – prior to the development of modern, efficient means of communication.

Medical textbooks often would carry very little information about individual rare conditions, and that which they did was frequently out of date and of little use when planning care and support for patients and their families. Redundant, obsolete or ineffective therapies would continue to be prescribed long after new knowledge had revealed them to be at best inappropriate, and at worst positively harmful.

Thanks to the internet, and due to a growing partnership between patient groups and expert specialist doctors, it is becoming increasingly feasible for clinicians and families to have access to good quality information about the care and management of a growing number of rare diseases.

There has been another interesting development too. Patient groups have used the internet to set up registers and to bring together resources located in far flung places to facilitate research and to create a more robust infrastructure for researchers to access, and to make developments sustainable over time rather than dependent on a series of short-term projects (as has often been the case in the past)!

### Tradition and Mindsets Coming Together

Unlike the USA, where access to health care tends to be based on individual entitlements, thereby creating a mindset that encourages rights based advocacy, the European solidarity-based systems have created a climate within which patients and families have tended to trust that, 'if something can be done it will be'. Whilst American patient groups will have lobbying and recourse to law to secure what they perceive as their rights at the forefront of their list of options, until recently at least, European groups have tended to see their role as complementary to that of the States.

While there was nothing much that could be done for children with serious diseases this reliance on the state health care system was probably OK – doctors did provide a degree of emotional support and organised palliation of symptoms. However, now there are possibilities for intervention (for some at least) and there is a growing realisation that, because of resource constraints, just because something can be done it doesn't mean that it will be. Parents of sick children in Europe are learning from their American cousins and are actively lobbying and campaigning at national and at European level for more research into treatments for childhood diseases, and for the rapid introduction of these novel therapies into clinical practice and their reimbursement by the state's health care system.

Thus, patient alliances such as EGAN (the European Genetic Alliances Network), Eurordis (European Organisation for Rare Disorders) and EACH (European Association for Children in Hospital) have been actively lobbying the European Commission and Parliament for the introduction of Regulations governing the development of paediatric medicines and paediatric focus of adult medicines. This lobbying has been in association with (but independent from) parallel initiatives by academic associations and industry bodies, all of whom want a clear framework within which they can work, and an appropriate range of incentives to encourage them to enter this field.

## Social Solidarity

Whilst the solidarity based health care systems of most European states have been one of their great strengths, in that all citizens have had access to a minimum standard of health care, rising demand is putting the consensus on which this provision is based and legitimated under increasing strain. Clearly, health care systems cannot afford to respond to patients' wants uncritically, but there is at present a poorly developed system for determining needs and the cost and clinical effectiveness of possible responses to these needs.

High-profile innovations, which tend to be expensive and which may only be useful for a small number of patients tend to attract the attention of service planners and those responsible for determining reimbursement policies. Long-established therapies often used by hundreds of thousands or millions of people do not attract attention and continue to be used, often at substantial cost to the health service, notwithstanding the fact that they may not work, deliver only a marginal benefit or have been superseded by newer, better medicines. Focussing attention on the innovative whilst turning a blind eye to the rest is inequitable, and will disproportionately impact on the likelihood of children getting access to the therapies that they need when these become available. As well as scrutinising new developments, evaluation should be extended across the health care spectrum and a disinvestment strategy introduced to stop paying for things that are of little use. This, if it were to be effectively introduced and policed, might help create the headroom for investment in novel medicines that deliver real health gain but which are beyond the reach of all but the wealthiest without the support of a solidarity-based health care system.

## Difficult Choices

We are all aware that medicines may have adverse effects. Therefore, although we are here to talk about medicines for children, we should also look at the health and treatment of children from a broader perspective. This is the reason why EGAN stresses the importance of early information, early diagnosis, prevention, informed reproductive choices and adequate preconception and prenatal care. More and more it becomes clear that the perinatal period, including the preconception phase, may have significant effects on child's future health. Environmental and lifestyle factors such as smoking, alcohol, use of medicines, diet, etc. are important. Genetic factors may also be important and without accurate, powerful diagnosis it can still happen that a second or third child with the same severe genetic disease is born in one family, either because the diagnosis in the first child was not made in time, or the diagnosis was made, but the treating physician did not inform the parents of the subsequent reproductive risks. EGAN's objective is healthy children, through the appropriate combination of preventative and therapeutic interventions in ways that reflect the needs of families and which are based on sound science – including safe, effective clinical trials that will produce innovative medicines for currently unmet medical needs.

Whilst animal-based research is a topic of increasing contention in many countries in Europe, with non-human primates being a source of particular concern to many, there can be little doubt about the importance of properly regulated research on animals in the search for therapies for the intractable disease of childhood.

Although such research makes us uncomfortable at times, and the search for replacements to animal-based work must go on, until effective models can be developed that mimic the human situation more closely than their animal counterparts the demand of parents for safe effective paediatric medicines must be respected. Nor should it be forgotten that animal-based research is not an end in itself (unless it is specifically targeted at the creation of veterinary medicines). Rather it is a step on the way to being able ethically to begin research in children – one that scientists and clinicians are anxious to achieve as quickly as possible, but not at the cost of jeopardising further the health of already vulnerable people. If you look at the propaganda put out by some of the opponents of animal-based work you could be led to believe that it is all cruel and heartless. Most is either not invasive or only minimally so, and although some does cause distress and suffering, this is kept to a minimum in responsible, regulated countries, and the animals euthanized afterwards.

Given a choice between my child and a mouse – or even a lot of mice – then most parents would opt for a chance for the child, and let the mice be used in research.

## From Hierarchy to Partnership

The traditional hierarchical model whereby 'doctor knows best' has crumbled, to be replaced by a partnership where parents are stakeholders alongside doctors, nurses, academics, drug companies, etc. in working out the best course of action to improve the outcomes for children with serious diseases. Indeed as children grow and mature, so they too are assuming a greater role in determining the best – or perhaps more often the least worst – way of managing their condition to produce the best possible quality of life.

Patient representatives are taking seats at the tables where decisions are made – not just as observers but as full partners with equal power to the others round the table. At the European Medicines Agency (EMEA), for example, patient representatives sit on the Management Board of the Orphan Medicinal Products Committee (COMP), they will have seats on the proposed Committee for Advanced Therapies (CAT) and also the Paediatric Committee and are engaging in many other ways with the work of that agency. Similar developments are taking place at national level. In the UK patient representatives are included on committees of the Department of Health such as the Genetics Commissioning Advisory Committee (GenCAG) and the UK Genetic Testing Network Steering Committee. They are also appearing on the committee of trade associations and professional bodies such as the UK's Medical Royal

Colleges. Similar examples can be found in many other European Countries.

Nor is patient participation confined to membership of committees, important though this is. Patients are also active in lobbying and campaigning for changes in law at national and European level to promote opportunities for research into unmet medical needs, particularly when these affect children or young people who would otherwise be denied the opportunity to grow into adults and take their place in society alongside everyone else. Public awareness is also needed, so that the importance of such paediatric research and development is understood by those not generally affected, and researchers not put off by ill-informed comment that implies they are simply using children as 'guinea pigs'.

It is useful to contrast the approach of patient and family support organisations for children with serious life-limiting disorders to that taken by some consumer groups. Whilst the approach of the former is to try and stand alongside the research community, acting as a critical friend and being part of the process, the latter can sometimes seem to be taking a confrontational stance – stressing the risks, the danger and the problems and sometimes almost seeming to forget (or at least discount) the fact that everything in the garden is not rosy for those children if no research is carried out. Without progress then unmet medical needs will remain just that, and children who might otherwise have been treated will remain untreatable, with all that implies for them and their families.

Of course, paediatric medicine is not an issue that is only relevant to patient organizations. All parents want the best possible treatment for their children when they are sick. We should all be concerned about possible side effects of the current unlicensed and off-label use of medicines in children. Families are no longer willing to accept unquestioningly the fact that a substantial proportion of all medicines that are used in children have not been investigated properly. Instead of the current lack of standards, we need the highest scientific and ethical standards for paediatric research and treatment. Children need priority [Priority Medicines for the Citizens of Europe and the World. Geneva, WHO, 2004]. Much greater investment in the health of children is needed. Some of this may even produce savings later by the avoidance of some of the diseases that now occur during middle or old age.

## Patient Groups as a Resource

It is sadly still the case that many of the rare disorders that affect children are poorly understood by the academic and clinical community. There has been little research done, and often that which has been carried out as been disjointed, transient and of poor quality. Of course there has been much which is world class, but this tends to be focussed on certain high-profile diseases like cystic fibrosis or muscular dystrophy rather than some of the lesser known ones.

For those where little is known, families are often an invaluable repository of first hand information about the impact of the disease on them and their affected children. The intimate business of providing daily care to the sick child necessarily creates a store of knowledge and understanding that is invaluable if it can only be tapped into effectively. Not only do they have this store of information, given the opportunity families are eager to share it with anyone who will listen.

This experience can be invaluable in developing training for healthcare professionals, taking hindsight and turning it into a pro-active tool that will enable doctors and others to provide information and support based on what parents and children need and want to know, not what professionals think they ought to know. It can help deliver this in ways that are appropriate and user friendly too, making it more likely that it will be heard, understood and acted on.

It can also guide researchers, contributing positively to the design of experiments and clinical trials, to the selection of appropriate end points and the choice of relevant biomarkers and about the importance of quality of life markers as well as those which reflect physiological or structural changes in the child.

And finally parents can help promote awareness of the importance and value of novel therapies, once these are licensed, to those responsible for authorising the prescription and/or reimbursement of these drugs by national health care systems, making it more likely that the journey from 'scientific bright idea' to pills in patients will be rewarded by speedy transfer into clinical practice and equitable availability to all the children who need to benefit from the fruits of this research and development.

Parent and patient organizations have a vital role in medical research and development. Patient registries and bio banks, based on uniform diagnostic criteria, will speed up future clinical research, and stimulate awareness of research possibilities for neglected or rare diseases in academia and industry. Many patient organisations have appointed scientific officers to streamline fragmented research initiatives and to highlight the research needs of their members. Patients should be regarded as a partner in the process towards innovative medicines. Patient's involvement will help identify the real therapeutic needs, balance urgency, risks and benefits, shorten the recruitment period and increase retention in clinical trials, and function as the intermediary between medical science and industry, the child, his family and society. Consultation with patient organizations at the start of research with children, will have added value. Participation in trial committees encourages development of study protocols, case record forms and patient information sheets, defining quality of life endpoints, adverse event reporting, data confidentiality issues and dissemination of study results.

### Importance of Personalized Medicine and Long-Term Follow-Up

We should not be satisfied that a certain drug at a certain dosage is effective only in 2/3 of the children who take it, but ineffective in the remaining 1/3. Variables that may increase effectiveness, e.g. age, gender, ethnicity and genetic differences, should be taken into account in order to enhance the effectiveness of targeted interventions including novel medicines. The well-being of children must be our first priority before commercial and scientific interests.

We do not know the long-term effects of many medicines in children. Long-term studies should assess the possible effects in developing children. Public private partnerships should be set up to secure continuity for those follow-up studies.

The new regulations on paediatric medicine are an opportunity for the pharmaceutical industry. To prove that commercial research can be combined with the highest ethical standards and improve the health of children currently living with serious diseases, paediatric research requires the paediatrician, industry and parents working together for the well-being of the child. Patient organisations play an important role in bringing all these together in the interests of children today and in the future.

## Conclusion

There is an urgent need for novel therapies to be developed to help treat the unmet health needs of millions of sick children across the world today. Whilst research and development is going on it is nowhere near enough, and parents rightly demand that more attention is given to this issue.

Patient and family support groups have a key role to play in helping produce safe, effective and affordable paediatric medicines available to all who need them on a sustainable basis. They are partners in a multi-stakeholder, trans-national programme that must turn its focus on helping more parents of newborn babies to get the answer they hope for when they ask that first question 'Is my baby alright?'

Rose K, van den Anker JN (eds): Guide to Paediatric Clinical Research.
Basel, Karger, 2007, pp 25–32

........................

# Paediatric Drug Development – Historical Background of Regulatory Initiatives

*Hans Stötter*

Swissmedic, Berne, Switzerland

All new medicinal products undergo a scrutinised regulatory review process before marketing authorisation, and it is the role of regulatory authorities to ensure the safety and efficacy of marketed medicinal products. The licensing process was introduced in the USA in response to adverse drug reactions that affected children and adults as early as 1962 by the Kefauver-Harris amendment to the Food Drug and Cosmetic Act [1], and as an example for European countries by the European Directive harmonising requirements for marketing authorisations (1965) or the UK Medicines Act (1968) [2]. Since this time, before any medicine is authorised for use, the product must have undergone extensive testing including pre-clinical tests and clinical trials to ensure that it is safe, of high quality and effective. It should be remembered that all this was started after disasters, such as malformations caused by thalidomide or adverse drug reactions in the newborn, e.g. the grey baby syndrome due to chloramphenicol, had occurred. It is ironic that legislation introduced following therapeutic misadventures in the newborn and the developing fetus has failed to ensure that medicines used in paediatric patients are fully tested as it relates to efficacy and toxicity [3].

Medical treatment has made considerable progress since the 1960s. However, since no or insufficient data have been generated in paediatric populations, many medicinal products received marketing authorisation for use in adult patients only. Once a medicinal product is approved, it may be prescribed by a physician for any population or disease state desired. This off-label use (the use in this population is not described/recommended in the label) together with unlicensed use (the medicinal product has no marketing authorisation) is reported to be as high as 60% in paediatric patients and more than 90% of patients treated in paediatric intensive care units. And while off-label use is not illegal, there are many problems associated with it: (a) patients are on their own trial; (b) the prescriber has to take the burden with the associated risks of inefficacy and/or adverse reactions; (c) safety or efficacy data from this experience are not collected and not made available to the health practitioner, although potentially useful for other patients, and (d) suitable formulations for young children are not available. Recent studies have shown that many young children are prescribed tablets or capsules, even though they are too young to swallow them and they may choke [4].

Adverse drug reactions in paediatric populations in connection with off-label use have higher incidence and greater severity, and have been reported in various countries; in some cases these were clearly resulting from dosing errors [5, 6].

Drug toxicity in children can be different from that in adults [7]. Methaemoglobinaemia due to percutaneous absorption of aniline dyes in neonates was reported in 1886 and again became a problem after exposure to sulfonamides or nitrates [8, 9]. Toxic deaths in children and adults were reported in 1938 due to a liquid preparation of sulphanilamide with diethyleneglycol [10], and kernicterus in 1956 by use of sulphisoxazole in neonates due to displacement of protein-bound bilirubin [11]. Catastrophes in the past, with the use of medicinal products without proper information, have happened such as the 'grey baby syndrome' with Chloramphenicol [12], the 'gasping syndrome' in neonates due to the preservative benzylic acid [13], hepatic failure in children younger than 3 years after exposure to sodium valproate [14], and liver necrosis in adolescents when paracetamol was taken as an overdose or in combination with other hepatotoxic drugs or ethanol [15]. We certainly have enough data demonstrating that the paediatric population is a vulnerable one. The high attempted suicide rate after treatment with selective serotonin reuptake inhibitors in adolescents did not raise concern in the period 1990–1995 when at its peak, clearly demonstrating that safety information of unlabelled use is problematic [16]. In fact, this more recent problem became public knowledge only after a cohort study performed by the British Medicines and Healthcare products Regulatory Agency (MHRA) and a thorough meta-analysis of clinical trials in adolescents performed by the FDA.

This problematic situation for the paediatric population was addressed by the FDA in 1979 by adding a paediatric subsection, in 1994 by adding a paediatric labelling requirement, in 1997 by the FDA modernisation act (FDAMA, section 111) which introduced exclusivity incentives, and in 1998 by paediatric study requirements (Pediatric Rule). The incentives were followed in 1999 by the Pediatric Exclusivity Provision, which led to the 2002 Best Pharmaceuticals for Children Act (BPCA). The paediatric rule was recently replaced by the Pediatric Research Equity Act (PREA, 2003). The incentive offered (6-month exclusivity for the active substance) and the funding for studies of off-patent products were highly appreciated by industry; however, the Pediatric Rule of 1998 was not. This rule was set up to avoid that manufacturers of new drugs limit their paediatric development to those drugs that will produce the greatest benefits, but instead to develop those which are most needed by children. While the 'carrot' was unanimously taken up, the 'stick' was not. A lawsuit challenging the Pediatric Rule was filed by three conservative groups, including the Competitive Enterprise Institute. In 2002, a USA district court judge ruled that the FDA lacked the legal authority to issue its 1998 Pediatric Rule: 'FDA's expansive interpretation of the Food Drug and Cosmetic Act lacks firm support in both law and tradition.' And Sam Kazman, general counsel to the Competitive Enterprise Institute said 'In our view the paediatric rule constituted a drastic change in the drug approval process'. These citations make it very clear that FDA's initiatives created a new task and responsibility for a regulatory authority: a request for studies in a paediatric population where the drug may be required was issued, instead of just evaluating data that were sent for review with a new drug application. But the FDA only had lost a battle, since in 2003 this new competence was given back to them by the House of Representatives who passed the bill to codify the new paediatric rule (Pediatric Research Equity Act, PREA). The FDA now has statutory authority to require pharmaceutical companies to test their products in children and has an enforcement authority for action in court when a company fails to submit a required paediatric assessment. This covers new medicinal products. For any new medicinal product, the manufacturer has to include paediatric studies in a marketing application unless a waiver or deferral has been obtained. Before the FDA can take action, the manufacturer has the opportunity to conduct paediatric studies voluntarily and earn 6 months of exclusivity. For old medicinal products, the FDA defines the requirements for paediatric studies: in cases (a) when there is a compelling need defined as the drug or biological product offers a meaningful therapeutic benefit and absence of labelling poses a risk, or (b) there is 'substantial use' and the absence of labelling poses a risk. Meaningful therapeutic benefit was defined as a significant improvement in the treatment, diagnosis, or prevention of a disease, compared to marketed products adequately labelled for that use in the relevant paediatric population. Such a benefit would be expected in a class of drugs or for an indication for which there is a need for additional therapeutic options. Substantial use was defined as more than 50,000 patients for the labelled indication.

There is international consensus regarding what kind of studies will be required in developing a medicinal product for use in the paediatric population. The International Conference on Harmonization (ICH), a joint effort of regulatory authorities and industry of USA, EU and Japan has finalised and implemented a guidance document in 2000 that describes the type and timing of paediatric studies (E11 Clinical Investigations of medicinal products in the paediatric population) [17]. This guidance document is accepted worldwide, so that development of medicinal products for use in children should follow the same rules.

In terms of clinical research, 'children' cannot be considered a single population (consider a premature newborn as compared to a 15-year-old). Therefore, studies may be more complex than studies in adults. Specific studies may be required in selected paediatric populations such as preterm, term newborns, infants, children or adolescents. In many cases data may be extrapolated from other populations such as adults or older age groups. The number of children suffering from specific diseases is generally lower than the number of adults and, the size of the respective populations having the disease may be less than the threshold for orphan designation. For this and other reasons, the European orphan drug Regulation has not been sufficient to deal with this situation.

In a publication on 120 new substances authorised from January 1995 to May 2001 by EMEA, 70 (58%) were of potential use in children [18]. Of these only 17 were authorised for all and 15 for some paediatric age groups. The majority (54%) were not appropriately tested in paediatric age groups. The proportion of drugs for which full paediatric labelling was available has not increased over time and, obviously, neither the increased number of publications on this issue nor the ICH guidance had any effect in absence of any incentives or rules.

However, the fact that in the USA the regulatory approval process encourages and rewards pharmaceutical sponsors to investigate drugs and biologics in children and to provide such information in the new drug application submission has been a great incentive for paediatric research in the USA. The numerous studies performed have produced data on pharmacokinetics in majority, and to a lesser extent on pharmacodynamics. Thus, the knowledge about drug metabolism in paediatric populations has increased. However, there is still a dearth of information on the basic mechanisms responsible for pharmacokinetics and pharmacodynamics, and the knowledge on ontogeny of drug biotransformation pathways, drug transport systems and pharmacologic receptor function, regulation and gene expression is at best rudimentary.

Innovative medicines can and do save lives, and the children of Europe deserve at least the same access to such innovation as that enjoyed by adults.

On September 29, 2004, the European Commission adopted a proposal for a Regulation of the Council and of the Parliament on Medicinal Products for Paediatric Use that aims to address the current situation. This proposal followed extensive research and consultation on possible solutions to this public health issue, and was supported by an 'Extended Impact Assessment' of the social and economic effects of the proposals on children and their families, healthcare professionals, industry and governments. The results of the 'Extended Impact Assessment' show that the proposal would lead to the availability of more and better medicines for children and that the pharmaceutical industry would benefit through incentives, encouraging innovation. This proposal has passed the European Parliament and Council in two successive readings. The latest proposal (Council common position) can be found at: http://europa.eu.int/eur-lex/lex/JOHtml.do?uri=OJ:C:2006:132E:SOM:EN:HTML. It is expected that this Regulation will enter into force by end of

2006 and will be immediately implementable by all 25 Member States of the European Union.

The European Regulation on better medicines for children deals with two scenarios concerning newer medicines, still under patent protection on the one hand, and older medicinal products which are unprotected on the other hand. This program is a composition of incentives and obligations. The key objectives of the Regulation are (1) to increase the development of and information on medicinal products for the paediatric population; (2) to increase marketing authorisations of medicines for use in children, and (3) to ensure that children's medicines are subject to high-quality research and children are not subjected to unnecessary clinical trials.

The EMEA Paediatric Committee will give proactive advice on development and also make decisions influencing drug development. It is clear that by taking responsibility for a medical minority such as the paediatric population, regulatory authorities acquire an additional competence and face new challenges. They give advice on the basis of existing data, request studies where they see a need, and give input into the development plan.

This new task requires regulatory authorities to use the available professional knowledge, to define where and when data are required and which type of data will be sufficient. This also requires a more intense interaction between industry, academia and regulatory authorities.

Early accessibility to study data and worldwide-shared information on details of studies performed in paediatric patients (also if negative) are needed to save this sensitive population from unnecessary clinical studies. This requires close collaboration and data exchange (including negative data) between data centres, study groups and regulatory authorities; paediatricians should be asked about their needs and also patients' disease groups should give their input.

Thus, procedures for paediatric marketing authorisations are far more complex than they used to be. They require more resources, and a knowledge-based network. In parallel to the European Commission and Council initiative, in 2001 the Committee for Medicinal products for Human use (CHMP, formerly CPMP) has set up a paediatric expert group (PEG) with the objectives to obtain information on medicinal products currently used in children, and agree where there are medical needs for the paediatric population, to contribute to guidelines relating to the development of medicinal products for paediatric use, define means and ways to make the information on paediatric medicinal products available to health care professionals and the general public, and to advise the European Commission on matters relating to paediatric medicines. The PEG has produced several guidance documents in particular on developing medicines for newborns (renal, liver, heart and lung immaturity), a population where clinical trials are especially difficult to perform, on paediatric formulations and on clinical trials in small populations. Paediatric needs have been evaluated in the areas of gastro-enterology, hepatology, anti-HIV products, pain treatment, rheumatology, oncology, immunology, cardiovascular, and central nervous system medicines. This work is done in close collaboration with the relevant learned societies at the European level. The PEG is also paving the way to establish the paediatric research network foreseen in the proposed Regulation.

At present, industry is not submitting all of the clinical studies requested by the FDA to other regulatory authorities. It is expected that the future European legislation will correct the situation. Global development should be an objective when it comes to paediatric and orphan medicines.

## References

1   1962 amendment of the Food Drug and Cosmetic Act (FDCA). http://www.mca.gov.uk/aboutagency/regframework/regframework.htm
2   Impicciatore P, Choonara I: Status of new medicines approved by the European Medicines Evaluation Agency regarding paediatric use. Br J Clin Pharmacol 1999;48:15–18.
3   Conroy S, Choonara I, Impicciatore P, Impicciatore P, Mohn A, Arnell H, Rane A, Knoeppel C, Seyberth H, Pandolfini C, Raffaelli MP, Rocchi F, Bonati M, t'Jong G, de Hoog M, van den Anker JN: Survey of unlicensed and off label drug use in paediatric wards in European countries. BMJ 2000;320:79–97.
4   Schirm E, Tobi H, de Vries TW, Choonara I, De Jong-van den Berg LTW: Lack of appropriate formulations of medicines for children in the community. Acta Paediatr 2003;92:1486–1489.
5   Impicciatore P, Choonara I, Clarkson A, Provasi D, Pandolfini C: Incidence of adverse drug reactions in paediatric in/out patients: a systematic review and meta-analysis of prospective studies. Br J Clin Pharmacol 2001;52:77–83.
6   Kozer E, Scolnik D, Keays T, Shi K, Luk T, Koren G: Large errors in the dosing of medicines for children. N Engl J Med 2002;346:1175–1176.
7   Choonara I, Rieder MJ: Drug toxicity and adverse drug reactions in children: a brief historical review. Paed Perinatal Drug Ther 2002;5:12–18.

8  Harry JW, Keitt AS: Studies on the efficacy and potential hazards of methylene blue therapy in aniline-induced methaemoglobinaemia. Br J Haematol 1983;54:29–41.

9  Comby HH: Cyanosis in infants caused by nitrates in well water. JAMA 1987;257: 2788–2792.

10  Geiling EMK, Cannon PR: Pathologic effects of elixir of sulphanilamide (diethylen glycol) poisoning. JAMA 1938;111:919–926.

11  Silverman WA, et al: A difference in mortality rate and incidence of kernicterus among premature infants allotted to two prophylactic antibacterial regimens. Pediatrics 1956; 18:614–624.

12  Weiss CF, Glazko AJ, Weston JK: Chloramphenicol in the newborn infant. N Engl J Med 1960;262:787–794.

13  Menon PA, Thach BT, Smith CH, Landt M, Roberts JL, Hillmann RE, et al: Benzyl alcohol toxicity in a neonatal intensive care unit. Am J Perinatol 1984;1:288–292.

14  Fisher E, Siemes H, Pund R, Wittfoht W, Nau H: Valproate metabolites in serum and urine during antiepileptic therapy in children with infantile spasms: abnormal metabolite pattern associated with reversible hepatotoxicity. Epilepsia 1992;33:165–171.

15  American Academy of Pediatrics: Acetaminophen toxicity in children. Pediatrics 2001;108:1020–1024. http://medicines.mhra.gov.uk/ourwork/monitorsafequalmed/safetymessages/ssrioverview_101203.htm

16  Brent DA: Antidepressants and pediatric depression: the risk of doing nothing. N Engl J Med 2004;351:1598–1601. http://www.fda.gov/cder/pediatric/

17  International Conference on Harmonization ICH: Guideline E11: Clinical investigation of medicinal products in the paediatric population. 19 July 2000. Available from: http://www.emea.eu.int/pdfs/human/ich/271199en.pdf

18  t'Jong GW, Stricker BHCh, Choonara I, van den Anker JN: Lack of effect of the European guidance on clinical investigation of medicines in children. Acta Paediatr 2002; 91:1233–1238.

Rose K, van den Anker JN (eds): Guide to Paediatric Clinical Research.
Basel, Karger, 2007, pp 33–37

......................

# ICH E 11: Clinical Investigation of Medicinal Products in the Paediatric Population

## The International Guidance on Clinical Drug Development in Children

*Klaus Rose*[a]    *Hans Stötter*[b]

[a]Pediatrics, F. Hoffmann-La Roche Ltd., Pharmaceuticals Division, Basel;
[b]Swissmedic, Berne, Switzerland

The International Conference on Harmonisation (ICH) [1] was established in 1990 as an initiative of the regulatory agencies and the pharmaceutical industry associations of the European Union, Japan and the United States of America. Since drug development by pharmaceutical companies had become increasingly international, a worldwide consensus on procedures was felt necessary. By ICH various guidance documents covering quality (Q), safety (S), efficacy (E) and multidisciplinary issues (M) have been created for worldwide submission [2]. Examples of such guidance documents in the efficacy section are ICH E 6 on good clinical practice, ICH E 5 on ethnicity, and ICH E 7 on studies in support of special populations: geriatrics. Drug development in children was felt important enough by the ICH to be taken up as a topic in 1998, and ICH E 11 [3] was written under the leadership of Steven Spielberg, at that time head of paediatric pharmacology in industry and currently Dean of Dartmouth Medical School [4]. It was adopted in 2000 by the regulatory agencies of Europe, Japan, USA, by Canada and Switzerland (both have observer status in the ICH), and Australia. ICH E 11 became a most valuable instrument in designing paediatric clinical research worldwide just in time, while initiatives of regulatory authorities gave a push to paediatric development. After a short introduction ICH E 11 gives guidance on various topics which will be briefly summarized.

## Introduction

The introduction addresses general principles that are still valid today. The pharmaceutical industry is addressed as follows:

*'Pediatric patients should be given medicines that have been appropriately evaluated for their use. Safe and effective pharmacotherapy in pediatric patients requires the timely development of information on the proper use of medicinal products in pediatric patients of various ages and, often, the development of pediatric formulations of those products.'*

While these lines address mainly pharmaceutical industry, the following lines involve all of us:

*'Obtaining knowledge of the effects of medicinal products in pediatric patients is an important goal. However, this should be done without compromising the well-being of pediatric patients participating in clinical studies. This responsibility is shared by companies, regulatory authorities, health professionals, and society as a whole.'*

In addition to industry, academia has a great task to deliver. Paediatric development can now be enforced by the FDA and this will be also the case in Europe now the EU regulation has been finalised. Not all studies from the USA have led to a change in paediatric labelling and in the future industry and health authorities will need to improve their dialogue with the aim to design better studies.

## Timing of General Paediatric Drug Development

*'Justification for the timing and the approach to the clinical program needs to be clearly addressed with regulatory authorities at an early stage and then periodically during the medicinal product development process. The pediatric development program should not delay completion of adult studies and availability of a medicinal product for adults.'*

A paediatric development plan is an absolute requirement in the USA today and will have to be presented in the EU as part of all submission for marketing authorization, for marketed products as well as for new medicinal products. Lack of data will need to be justified.

## Paediatric Formulations

The need for paediatric formulations is emphasized to allow accurate dosing and improve patient compliance. International harmonization on the acceptability of excipients would be desirable.

## Timing of Clinical Studies

Drug development in the paediatric population should be started early. With respect to timing the guideline distinguishes:
- *'Medicinal products intended to treat serious or life-threatening diseases, occurring in both adults and pediatric patients, for which there are currently no or limited therapeutic options.' 'Drug development should begin early in the pediatric population, following assessment of initial safety data and reasonable evidence of potential benefit. Pediatric study results should be part of the marketing application database.'*
- *'Other diseases and conditions.' 'Testing of these medicinal products in the pediatric population would usually not begin until phase 2 or 3. In most cases, only limited pediatric data would be available at the time of submission of the application, but more would be expected after marketing.'*

## Types of Studies

As a consequence of the new regulation, recruitment of children in various age groups into pharmacokinetic and pharmacodynamic studies will further increase in the USA and Europe. Principles are laid down in ICH E 11 when pharmacokinetic/pharmacodynamic studies may suffice for submission of a paediatric indication or a new galenical form suitable to treat small children. It is also pointed out that emphasis should be given to develop appropriate age-specific surrogate markers/endpoints and novel technologies for assessment, e.g. bloodless procedures. Scientific advice procedures are in place for interaction between industry and regulatory authorities on those issues.

---

'When novel indications are being sought for the medicinal product in pediatric patients, or when the disease course and outcome of therapy are likely to be different in adults and pediatric patients, clinical efficacy studies in the pediatric population would be needed.'

Four types of studies are discussed in detail and just the major points are highlighted here: (1) Pharmacokinetic studies should be generally conducted in patients, not healthy volunteers; the volume of blood withdrawn needs to be minimized, bioavailability studies should be conducted in adults whenever appropriate. (2) Efficacy studies: it may be necessary to develop distinct clinical endpoints/surrogate markers differing from those in adults. (3) Safety studies: extra attention should be given to possible late adverse events. Sponsors should consider effects on skeletal, behavioral, cognitive, sexual, and immune maturation and development. (4) Postmarketing studies: might be necessary in some cases.

### Age Groups

'Any classification of the pediatric population into age categories is to some extent arbitrary, but a classification such as the one below provides a basis for thinking about study design in pediatric patients. Decisions on how to stratify studies and data by age need to take into consideration developmental biology and pharmacology. Thus, a flexible approach is necessary to ensure that studies reflect current knowledge of pediatric pharmacology. The identification of which ages to study should be medicinal product-specific and justified.'

Five age categories are described by depicting the specific problems in a certain age group: preterm newborn infants, term newborn infants (0–27 days), infants and toddlers (28 days to 23 months), children (2–11 years), and adolescents (12 to 16–18 years, depending on region). Obviously as stated above, current knowledge on pharmacokinetics and the specific data of a certain compound have to be considered in the decision on age groups.

## Ethical Issues

Children are a vulnerable population. The role of IRB/EC (Institutional Review Board/Ethical Committee) is critical to the protection of the study participants. Recruitment must be free from inappropriate inducement, and any compensation needs to be reviewed by IRB/EC. Although the child is legally unable to provide informed consent and the parents have to give the consent on its behalf, children of appropriate intellectual maturity should in addition give assent by a signature of their own. A participating child's wish to withdraw from the study must be respected. Studies in handicapped or institutionalized children should be limited to diseases found principally in these populations. Every effort must be made to anticipate and minimize risks in paediatric trials, and mechanisms need to be in place to ensure that a study can be rapidly terminated should an unexpected risk be noted. Invasive procedures must be minimized, and the study personnel must be specially trained. The number of acceptable venipunctures needs to be clearly limited in the protocol.

## Conclusion

ICH E 11 has the scope to facilitate and improve data generation for use of medicinal products in children and gives guidance on drug development for paediatric populations. It documents the strong commitment of both regulatory authorities and pharmaceutical industries that children should be allowed to benefit from improvements of pharmacotherapy, with a careful balance between risks and benefits.

## References

1   The International Conference on Harmonisation of Technical Requirements for Registration of Pharmaceuticals for Human Use, www.ich.org
2   ICH Information Brochure, http://www.ich.org/LOB/media/MEDIA410.pdf
3   Clinical Investigation of Medicinal Products in the Pediatric Population, http://www.ich.org/LOB/media/MEDIA487.pdf
4   http://dms.dartmouth.edu/dean/sps_background.shtml

Rose K, van den Anker JN (eds): Guide to Paediatric Clinical Research.
Basel, Karger, 2007, pp 38–46

··············

# Ethical Challenges of Clinical Research in Children

## Protection from Risks vs. Access to Benefits

*David Neubauer*[a]  *Pirjo Laitinen-Parkkonen*[b]  *Dirk Matthys*[c]

[a]University Children's Hospital Ljubljana, Department of Child,
Adolescent and Developmental Neurology, Ljubljana, Slovenia;
[b]National Agency for Medicines, Helsinki, Finland;
[c]Department of Pediatrics, Ghent University, Ghent, Belgium

### General Considerations

The twin studies in Birkenau and other 'research projects' during the Nazi regime in Germany resulted in the Nuremberg Principles of Research Ethics [1]. The major aim of the Nuremberg code was protection of the vulnerable subjects. However, the first principle ('the voluntary consent of the human subject is absolutely essential') makes paediatric research virtually impossible. Despite the Nuremberg code, in the 1950s and early 1960s a number of studies were performed on institutionalised children: at Willowbrook State School, New York, mentally retarded children were infected with the hepatitis virus to study the natural history of the disease. This is 1 of the 22 research projects Beecher [2] reported as being unethical.

In the 1970s special attention was paid to the vulnerability of the child. Protection from risks generated by research was prominent: The World Medical Association Declaration of Helsinki 1964 (last amend-

P.L.-P. contributed to this chapter only as an individual expert, and does not represent the CHMP. The views expressed here are her personal views and may not be understood or quoted as being made on behalf of the CHMP or reflecting the position of the CHMP.

ment Tokyo, 2004) [3] provides the ethical principles for medical research involving human subjects. Special attention is paid to the 'legally incompetent minor' who should 'not be included in research unless the research is necessary to promote the health of the population represented and this research cannot instead be performed on legally competent persons'.

Another landmark in ethical guidelines is the Belmont report of 1979 [4]: it summarizes the basic ethical principles identified by The National Commission for the Protection of Human Subjects of Biomedical and Behavioural Research. Those 3 basic ethical principles are respect for persons, beneficence and justice. Respect for persons means protection of those with diminished autonomy. Children clearly belong to the group of persons that requires extensive protection.

It is obvious that ethical guidelines are essential, but the exclusion of children from research resulted in Shirkey's statement in 1963 that children are becoming 'therapeutic orphans' [5]. The Convention on the Rights of the Child, adopted by the United Nations General Assembly in 1989, stipulates that 'Children have the right to the highest attainable level of health' [6]. Children should be protected from risks but must have access to benefits from research. Medical research involving children is essential for the improvement of care [7]. In the 1970s, P. Ramsey was definitely opposed to non-therapeutic research or research without direct benefit to the child. Nowadays, the majority of paediatric researchers are convinced that the distinction between therapeutic and non-therapeutic research is artificial. The aim of a research project is to obtain generalised knowledge of vital importance.


### Placebo-Controlled Clinical Trials in Children

The issue of testing medications in children still presents a dilemma. We should remember some of the tragedies from the past, especially those connected with sulfanilamide-treated deaths [8] and the epidemic of birth defects associated with thalidomide which were the cause of most of the changes regarding law and regulations that govern the testing and marketing of new drugs [9, 10]. However, the testing of medications for safety and efficacy has mainly benefited adults (who offer larger cohorts and definitely take more medications than children), while medications used by children are rarely tested on them and even more – unapproved or unlicensed and 'off-label' drugs are often used in children's hospitals [11]. Also, a considerable number of drugs prescribed in general practice are not licensed for use in children or are prescribed off label and the absolute number of children using such drugs is much higher than in a clinical care setting. This situation is highly unsatisfactory and efforts should be made to improve it [12]. On the other hand, since 1997 there has been an astounding progress in the amount of the paediatric clinical trials and it is likely that today tens of thousands of children are participating in studies of medications that are funded by industry or by the governments [10]. Recent and very important instruments are the documents issued by the 1990 funded International Conferences of Harmonization (ICH).[1] The first principle of ICH states: 'Clinical trials should be conducted in accordance with the ethical principles that have the origin in the Declaration of Helsinki and that are consistent with Good Clinical Practice and the applicable requirements.'[2]

## Current Issues

Despite legislative obstacles other obstacles also exist which may seem difficult to solve – the ethical issues, off-label prescribing practice, investment and clinical doability/feasibility [13]. Under the regulations children are considered a vulnerable group and as such require additional protection as research subjects and there are recent papers developed within the Working group of Ethics, Confederation of European Specialists in Paediatrics/European Academy of Paediatrics (CESP/ EAP) dealing with these issues [14–20]. Despite the additional regulations for children they may not be adequately protected in practice [14]. Because of possible different explanations of what is the risk and what

---

[1] All these documents can be found at the ICH website at: www.ich.org.
[2] A revised version of the Declaration of Helsinki was issued in October 2000 and it remains a vital expression of medical ethics whose aims deserve unanimous support. Section 29 in particular states that 'The benefits, risks, burdens and effectiveness of a new method should be tested against those of the best current prophylactic, diagnostic and therapeutic methods. This does not preclude the use of placebo or no treatment in studies where no proven prophylactic, diagnostic or therapeutic method exists.' See this and other relevant documents at the EMEA website at: http://www.emea. eu.int/.

**Table 1.** Classification of paediatric research [adapted from ref. 10]

| Category | Requirements for approval by the institutional review board |
|---|---|
| Research not involving greater than minimal risk | adequate provisions for soliciting the assent of children and the permission of their parents or representatives |
| Research involving greater than minimal risk but presenting the prospect of direct benefit to individual subjects | risk justified by anticipated benefit to subjects; ratio of anticipated benefit to risk is at least as favourable as that for available alternative |
| Research involving greater than minimal risk and no prospect of direct benefit to individual subjects, but likely to yield generalisable knowledge about the subject's disorder or condition | risk represents minor increase over minimal risk; intervention or procedure presents experiences reasonably commensurate with those inherent in subjects' actual or expected medical, dental, psychological, social, or educational situations; research likely to yield generalisable knowledge about the subject's disorder or condition that is of vital importance for the understanding or amelioration of it |
| Research not otherwise approvable that presents an opportunity to understand, prevent, or alleviate a serious problem affecting the health and welfare of children | institutional review board of the Department of Health and Human Services, after consultation with panel experts, must find that the research presents a reasonable opportunity to meet criteria and will be conducted in accord with sound ethical principles |

are the benefits of all research involving children (and especially what are the differences of such studies with regard to the studies in adults) some federal regulations were proposed in the USA which apply to research conducted or funded by the Department of Health and Human services or regulated by FDA (table 1) [10, 21]. However, as has already been stated, focusing only on national instruments such as these regulations will not provide sufficient protection for all our children and an international ethical framework supported by international sharing of data would be an ideal model [22].

## Pros and Cons of Placebo-Controlled Trials in Children

The use of placebo has been considered by many as non-realistic and unjustified. Strict interpretation of a revised version of Declaration of Helsinki (see footnote [2]) would appear to rule out those randomised-controlled trials (RCTs) that use a placebo (that is a dummy treatment administered to control group children) whenever licensed therapeutic method already exists, and thus preferring active controls. However, although the efficacy of some new medicinal products can be satisfactory demonstrated without the use of placebo, for others judicious use of placebo remains essential to demonstrate the efficacy and safety of the product. There are many groups of therapeutic agents where placebo controls are justified and even mandatory: analgesics, many psychopharmacological drugs, antihypertensives, antiarrhythmics and many drugs used in primary prevention. There are number of conditions which should be taken into account when considering use of placebo-controlled trials. It is essential that the use of placebo does not pose a risk of serious discomfort, irreversible harm or death to the child or that existing therapy improves survival or decreases serious morbidity. Also, the child included in the trial (and his/her legal representative) must receive and understand appropriate information on the trial and give informed written consent/assent [15–17, 20]. The child's (and his/her representative's) right is to withdraw at any time but still receive conventional treatment and this should strictly be respected. In all EU (and other foreign countries) similar ethical and Good Clinical Practice standards should be applied for trials performed. These aspects should fall within the responsibilities of ethics committees reviewing protocols of clinical trials in children.[3] Forbidding placebo-controlled trials in therapeutic areas where there are proven prophylactic, diagnostic or therapeutic methods would preclude obtaining reliable scientific evidence for the evaluation of the benefits and risks of new medicinal products, and be contrary to public health interest as there is a need for both new products and alternatives to existing medicinal products.

[3] 'The accepted basis for the conduct of clinical trials in humans is founded in the protection of human rights and dignity of the human being with regard to the application of biology and medicine, as for instance reflected in the Helsinki Declaration' and 'A clinical trial may be initiated only if the Ethics Committee and/or the competent authority comes to the conclusion that the anticipated therapeutic and public health benefits justify the risks and may be continued only if compliance with this requirement is permanently monitored.' See: EMEA/17424/01.

## Ethical Considerations on Randomised-Controlled Paediatric Trials

Evidence-based medicine (EBM) is the conscientious, explicit, and judicious use of current best evidence in making decisions about the care of individual patients. The practice of EBM means integrating individual clinical expertise with the best available external evidence from systematic research. Best available external clinical evidence means clinically relevant research, often from the basic sciences of medicine, the power of prognostic markers, precision of diagnostic tests and the efficacy and safety of therapeutic, rehabilitative and preventive regimens. In the health sciences there are various study designs and regarding their impact they are classified as meta-analyses, RCTs (randomised-controlled clinical trials), cohort studies, case-control studies, case reports, non-systematic reviews and cost-effectiveness analyses. To find out about the accuracy of a diagnostic test we need to find proper cross-sectional studies of patients on randomised trials, for a question of prognosis we need proper follow-up studies, when asking questions about therapy we should try to avoid the non-experimental approaches since they may lead to false-positive conclusions about efficacy.

Recently, it has been proven that RCTs are the second-cited study design and are therefore the preferable way of research studies [23]. The majority of other studies have a similar impact, while case reports do not bare many citations if any. On the other hand, it has been stated that the proportion of most frequently cited articles funded by industry is significantly ($p = 0.001$) increasing over time and is sometimes even exclusive [24]. This implies that the future research (also in the paediatric field of research) will be mostly focused on the industry-funded RCTs. There were some doubts about the properly designed RCTs in certain conditions as some trials could be too small and too poorly designed to be able to detect or to refute reliably realistically modest but clinically important benefits or hazards of treatment, and that limited funding for research and unfamiliarity with issues of consent may be important obstacles [25]. The methodological concerns can also be a major reason for the acceptance or refusal of certain studies and the validity of a test can be one of its most important contributes as well as there may be demanding high levels of proof before funding is approved. However, even in common disorders there can be embarrassingly few data and this would create a catch-22 situation [26]. In paediatrics, we lack long-term population studies to demonstrate the balance of benefits versus side effects. It is rather unlikely to set up a long-term RCT with placebo controls because not many parents want to risk their child being in the placebo arm. To emulate the success of certain fields, such as paediatric oncology (where in many countries most children are in some kind of study even if simply an observational one), requires an infrastructure as well as willpower and enormous resources [26].

However, some questions about therapy do not require RCTs or cannot wait for the trials to be conducted and if this is so, we must follow the trail to the next best external evidence and work from there [27, 28]. There are probably few childhood syndromes for which there are sufficient numbers of participants on which to perform RCT [29]. As the result of the increase in good paediatric studies, the investigators and instructional review boards may gain paediatric expertise as well and we should hope that the increased participation of children in clinical trials based on good clinical practice recommendations [15–19] will continue.

Finally, we should be aware that in cases where there is a limited number of evaluable subjects (which is frequently the case in paediatrics) the importance of collecting maximum information from the cases observed becomes essential, especially if the only data available consist of a series of isolated clinical information. Standardised analysis of information from various sources and on the basis of objective criteria would be of potential interest in the absence of other methods of evaluation.

## Conclusion

We hope that in the future the major obstacles regarding the problems in paediatric drug development (limitation of the size, limitation of those willing to participate, either as placebo or healthy controls, limitation of doctors willing to take part in clinical trials, limitations by too strict criteria – for inclusion or exclusion) will soon be removed and that paediatricians will not be forced to adopt extraordinary measures to insure that their patients are not harmed by treatments that have not been adequately studied in children [30]. Finally, most important is the recognition of all different parties involved that it is in the interest of children to evaluate medicinal products with scientifically proven methods, if possible by paediatric placebo-controlled trials, which should only be justified when their design, enrolment and conduct ensure that they really address the best interests of the children-participants with a view to their health and a concern of their dignity.

## References

1   The Nuremberg Code: www.ushmm.org/research/doctors/codeptx.htm
2   Beecher HK: Ethics and clinical research. N Engl J Med 1966;274:1354–1360.
3   The World Medical Association Declaration of Helsinki 1964: www.wma.net/e/policy/b3.htm
4   The Belmont Report: http://ohsr.od.nih.gov/guidelines/belmont.html
5   Shirkey HC: Editorial comment: therapeutic orphans. J Pediatr 1968;119:119–120.
6   General Assembly of the United Nations: Convention on the Rights of the Child, 20 November 1989. www.unicef.org/crc/crc.htm
7   Sauer PJJ: Research in children. A report of the Ethics Working Group of CESP. Eur J Pediatr 2002;161:1–5.
8   Anon: Elixir of sulfonamide-massengil: chemical, pharmacologic, pathologic and necropsy reports. Preliminary toxicity reports on diethylene glycol and sulfonamide. JAMA 1937;109:1531–1539.
9   Kauffman RE: Drug safety, testing, and availability for children. Child Legal Rights J 1998;18:27–34.
10  Steinbrook R: Testing medications in children. N Engl J Med 2002;347:1462–1470.
11  't Jong GW, Vulto AG, de Hoog M, Schimmel KJM, Tibbole D, van den Anker JN: Unapproved and off-label use of drugs in a children's hospital. N Engl J Med 2000; 343:1125.
12  't Jong GW, Eland IA, Stukenboom CJM, van den Anker JN, Stricker BHCh: Unlicensed and off label prescriptions of drugs to children: population based cohort study. BMJ 2002;324:1313–1314.
13  Ramet J: What the paediatricians need – the launch of paediatric research in Europe. Eur J Pediatr 2005;164:263–265.
14  Kurz R, Gill D, Mjones S: Ethics in the daily medical care of children. Statement of the Ethics WG of the CESP. Eur J Pediatr 2006;165:83–86.
15  Gill D, et al: Ethical principles and operational guidelines for good clinical practice in paediatric research. Recommendations of the Ethics WG of the CESP. Eur J Pediatr 2004;163:53–57.
16  Gill D, Ethics Working Group of the Confederation of European Specialists in Paediatrics: Guidelines for informed consent in biomedical research involving paediatric populations as research participants. Eur J Pediatr 2003;162:455–458.
17  Kurz R, Gill D: Practical and ethical issues in paediatric clinical trials. Appl Clin Trials 2002;11:60–63.
18  Sauer PJJ: Research in children. Eur J Pediatr 2002;161:1–5.
19  Kurz R, Crawley FP: The Clinical Trial Directive's ethical impact on research into diseases that cause incapacity and diseases of children: perspectives from non-commercially funded research in hospitals. Int J Pharm Med 2003;17:7–9.

20   De Lourdes Levy M, Larcher V, Kurz R, et al: Informed consent/assent in children. Eur J Pediatr 2003;162:629–633.

21   Steinbrook R: Improving protection for research subject. N Engl J Med 2002;346: 1838.

22   Crawley FP, Kurz R, Nakamura H: Testing medications in Children (reply). N Engl J Med 2003;348:763.

23   Patsopoulos NA, Analatos AA, Ioannidis JP: Relative citation impact of various study designs in the health sciences. JAMA 2005;293:2362–2366.

24   Patsopoulos NA, Analatos AA, Ioannidis JP: Origin and funding of the most frequently cited papers in medicine: database analysis. BMJ 2006;332:1061–1064.

25   Dickinson K, Bunn F, Wentz R, Edwards P, Roberts I: Size and quality of randomized controlled trials in head injury: review of published studies. BMJ 2000;320:1308–1311.

26   Baxter P: Evidence based medicine (editorial). DMCN 2004;46:723.

27   Sackett DL, Rosenberg WMC, Gray JAM, Haynes RB, Richardson WS: Evidence based medicine: what it is and what it isn't. BMJ 1996;312:71–72.

28   Draft Guideline on Clinical Trails in Small Populations, CHMP/EWP/83561/2005.

29   Ferrie CD, Livingstone JH: Epilepsy and evidence-based medicine: a vote of confidence in expert opinion from the National Institute of Clinical Excellence? DMCN 2005;47:204–206.

30   Groopman J: The Pediatric Gap. New Yorker 2005;80:32–37.

Rose K, van den Anker JN (eds): Guide to Paediatric Clinical Research.
Basel, Karger, 2007, pp 47–58

··············

# Consent and Assent in Paediatric Clinical Trials

*Jane Lamprill*[a]    *Patricia A. Fowler*[b]

[a]Paediatric Research Consultancy, Oxford, and [b]Harlow, UK

## Introduction

Consent and assent for children participating in paediatric clinical trials is a key issue in relation to the Paediatric Regulation for Medicinal Products in Children [1]. Pharmaceutical companies are now mandated to provide paediatric data for European regulatory submissions unless a waiver or deferral is agreed upon. More paediatric studies will be conducted and it is essential that the consent/assent process for paediatric clinical trials is well regulated and transparent [2].

## Definitions

Misunderstandings and abuse around definitions of consent, assent and acquiescence to research have led to law suits over the years where people have not realised that they were clinical trial participants, e.g. the Tuskegee study where Afro-Caribbean American males had treatment withheld to observe the development of syphilis [3]. Other research performed without consent resulted in the forming of the Nuremberg Code which states that 'The voluntary consent of the human subject is absolutely essential for their protection and to prevent harm' [4].

*Consent* means voluntary permission by one who has been informed in language they understand about the risks and benefits of the proposed research, and have legal authority to consent on their own behalf or for someone they have legal responsibility for, e.g., parent, guardian, legal representative. In a paediatric setting, a young person may sign his/her own consent form after reaching the age of legal majority, which varies internationally. *Assent* is the same informed voluntary permission but by someone having no legal authority, i.e. a child. 'Under-age' children may have legal rights to consent for themselves in special circumstances relating to medical treatment [5] but not for medicinal research within the remit of the EU Clinical Trials Directive [6]. For consent and assent to be valid they must be freely given and fully informed.

*Acquiescence* is a passive state of submission without questioning or protest. If a child or parent acquiesces to interventive biomedical research without fully informed and written consent/assent, the researcher has performed an illegal act and could be sued for 'trespass of the person'. Under European Directive 2001/20/EC [6], this could incur a prison sentence if considered gross misconduct. Sponsor companies would also be liable if research was not adequately monitored.

Consent is not a single response at the beginning of the study but 'needs a willing, ongoing commitment that may falter during a difficult project' [7]. This is true in paediatric trials where a parent and child may need a lot of support from the research team throughout a longitudinal study. If consent and assent are constantly considered, families feel less pressurised to participate. This usually assists with ongoing compliance.

*Voluntary participation:* As many children do not know what 'voluntary' means, a written and verbal explanation of this in simple terms is essential. Ethical difficulties around voluntariness also arise where the subject population is illiterate and financially disadvantaged. When healthcare requires payment, an impoverished mother may consent her child for research as her only route to a paediatrician. Clinically useful data may be gained, e.g., from blood tests but probably against the child's will as most small children are terrified of needles.

It is therefore an ethical imperative to provide study information in a form the parent and child can understand (e.g. pictures, audio), a clear explanation from the investigator and local anaesthetic cream available to minimise distress for invasive procedures.

## Refusing Assent (Dissent) and Alleviating Distress

Most guidance states that the refusal of the child to participate must be respected. However, Wendler [8] suggests that research staff should adopt a strategy of 'stop, assess and address'. At the first sign of distress and dissent the procedure should be stopped. A short pause to allow the child to feel in control, further explanation and an assessment of the situation may be all that is needed to reassure the child. E.g. a minor about to have a painless ECG may become distressed if they think electricity will be put *into* them, and can be reassured by a simple explanation. Often it is not the procedure they object to, but being restrained (e.g. arm held still for venipuncture) so again assent and dissent need to be assessed individually. Children may be distressed by separation anxiety if their parent is not with them during the procedure, or they may be anxious to avoid potential shame when asked to do something complicated if they have a very full bladder. Where research distress is temporary and the child is well prepared for the procedure, assent is not usually a problem – especially as children have been shown to perform research for altruistic reasons [9]. Wendler [8] is clear that should the child exhibit signs of inconsolable persistent distress the study should be stopped immediately. This is very important, for example, if a child is needle phobic. It would be very unethical to insist on a blood draw for research purposes as this could jeopardise future attempted health care provision [10].

## Country-Specific Requirements for the Consent/Assent Process

A global snapshot of some of these requirements has been summarised in table 1. This is believed to be correct at the time of writing. These are not comprehensive but will give some indication of local variability. Local laws should always be consulted, as should Ethics Committees (EC) or Independent Review Boards (IRB) as criteria may be decided on a case-by-case basis, and may change over time.

**Table 1.** Global snapshot of paediatric consent/assent requirements at June 2006

| Country | Legal age consent to research | How many parents/legal guardians give consent | Lower age for child assent |
|---|---|---|---|
| Australia | • 18 years<br>• occasionally a child under the age of 18 may be able to consent | • usually only one<br>• EC or sponsor may in rare circumstances require both | • no formal 'assent'<br>• it is at the investigator's discretion as to whether a child has sufficient capacity to read and sign a children's participant consent form aimed at the reading understanding of a 10-year-old |
| Czech Republic | • 18 years | • one parent | • when child is able to understand can either obtain assent or may countersign IC with parents (usually from age 12) |
| E. Africa | • over 18 years | • one (that has custody of the child) | • no official lower age but general practice is around 10 years |
| Estonia | • 18 years | • one parent | • no official lower age |
| France | • 18 years<br>• exceptionally 16 years for emancipated minor<br>• article 477 French civil code | • both holders of parental authority for unemancipated minor for biomedical research:<br>• one consent permitted under certain circumstances<br>• article L1122-2-11 French public health code | • assent actively sought<br>• age of assent when child can read and understand – usually 7 years<br>• refusal or revocation of consent cannot be ignored<br>• recommandation 8 of Déclaration politique de la FIP relative à la recherche pharmaceutique en pédiatrie |
| Germany | • 18 years | • both if both have right to care (this is determined at divorce) | • 6–8 years |
| Gulf State | • 18 years but EC or IRB may allow 16 years, depending on the trial | • both parents | • assent is not common<br>• all children under 18 will have the parents' consent |
| Ireland | • 18 years | • one parent | • not specified |

Lamprill/Fowler

**Table 1** (continued)

| Country | Legal age consent to research | How many parents/legal guardians give consent | Lower age for child assent |
|---|---|---|---|
| Israel | • 18 years | • both parents unless permission granted from EC for only one parent | • no official lower age although a child may be asked to add a signature to the parent consent form |
| Japan | • 20 years | • one parent or legal guardian | • no legal requirement for assent but MHLW require junior high school students and >13 years to sign assent form<br>• in practice children >7 years usually sign an assent form |
| Latvia | • 18 years | • one parent | • not specified |
| Lithuania | • 18 years | • strict requirement for both parents<br>• single mother can sign consent but must state her status on consent form<br>• if parents divorced stepfather may sign if he has official guardian rights | • no legal age<br>• ECs require subjects from 4 years of age to assent |
| Norway | • 16 years | • one parent | • assent according to age of understanding |
| Romania | • 18 years | • no explicit requirement<br>• ideally both but if divorced/single parent: adult with custody of child signs form | • no legal age of assent to research<br>• regulatory agency requires assent forms for children >12 years |
| Slovakia | • 18 years | • both parents | • at 6 (if they are able to read and understand) |
| Spain | • 18 years | • one parent | • from 12 till 18 years, subjects sign own assent form in addition to parental consent |
| Sweden | • 18 years | • both parents | • by law needed from 15 years |

Table 1 (continued)

| Country | Legal age consent to research | How many parents/legal guardians give consent | Lower age for child assent |
|---|---|---|---|
| Thailand | • age of general legal activity is 20 but<br>• RECs usually take 18 years as age of consent for research as hospitals have 18 as age of consent for treatment | • one parent can be the legal representative | • no legal requirement for age of assent<br>• some REC require >13 years to sign own assent form<br>• may vary from Institute to Institute |
| UK | • 16 years<br>• If child under 18 years refuses life-saving research drug (e.g. for cancer) then parent consent may over-ride dissent but court may have to decide | • one parent | • no lower limit defined but usually children of school age can assent for themselves in addition to parent consent<br>• assent flexible depending on Investigator opinion = usually decided on case by case basis<br>• UK regulatory guidance found at www.corec.org.uk/applicants/help/guidance.htm#consent<br>• separate information sheets required for children in language they can understand<br>• need translations for studies in ethnically diverse inner city areas<br>• COREC requirements for information sheets:<br>  • <5 years (simple words/pictures)<br>  • 6–12 years + assent form<br>  • 13–15 years + assent form<br>• suggest 'paediatric' subjects >16 years will need simpler information than parent version + easier language consent form or recruitment will be sub-optimal |
| USA | • varies from State to State<br>• usually 18 years<br>• NIH says 21 but State law usually prevails | • usually only one<br>• both parents must give consent if IRB considers study is > minimal risk with no benefit to child | • children required to sign assent form from the 'age of assent'<br>• age varies from IRB to IRB<br>• American Academy Pediatrics 1995 says it is 7 years<br>• most IRBs therefore say 7 but can be 10, 11 or 12 years |

## Main Factors Affecting Consent/Assent

*Timing*
- ICH/GCP [11] states that sufficient time should be allowed for a participation decision to be reached but is vague about how long this should be. The majority of ethics committees require an explanation if this is less than 24 h.
- Visits need to be timed conveniently for parents as the consent process should not be rushed. At least an hour may be required for discussion in terms the child and family can understand.
- Some studies involving serious disease require consent at or near diagnosis. This is extremely distressing for families and treatment will need rapid commencement. Great care should be taken in protocol planning – e.g could the child be started on supportive measures without risking harm – to give families more time to decide?

*Age of Child and Parent*
- *Child:* Research by Alderson [13] suggests that experience is more relevant than age for assent purposes, e.g. children as young as 5 who have had frequent orthopaedic surgery are more likely to understand their disease and hospital procedures well enough to desire involvement in decision-making processes about them.
- Age of assent has been widely debated. Seven years is recommended by the American Academy of Pediatrics (and by English King Edward III in the 12th century) but this varies from IRB to IRB. Interestingly, Wendler's [8] research suggests that it is not until 14 years of age that young people can fully grasp abstract concepts, i.e. 'moral reasons to help others independent of reward or punishment', reasons to participate, purpose of research and how the study 'pertains to their own circumstances'.
- If the child is a toddler they may have some understanding about what is required of them but of course will not have capacity to assent.
- *Parent:* There are many very young mothers (the UK has the highest teenage pregnancy rate in Europe). In one UK study, both the mother and the child were under 16 but both eligible for the same trial. They were happy to take part – so grandmother consented for them both. Local laws in other countries may vary.

- First-time parents may be inexperienced so consenting their young children, e.g. for a vaccine study where they are worried anyway, can be stressful. Information needs to be easy to read and understand and sufficient time allowed for talking through the project.

*Competency to Make Decisions*
- 'Many children are vulnerable, easily bewildered and frightened and unable to express their needs or defend their interests' [7].
- Decisions regarding competency need to be made by the investigator on a case-by-case basis and depend heavily on the parental knowledge of the child.
- Some children are very enthusiastic to participate but incompetent to decide for themselves because they don't understand the implications of what will happen to them.
- Competence to make decisions develops with increasing autonomy – teenagers prefer to make their own decisions. However, they will still need subtle support and information sheets suited to their age group.
- A big problem being addressed by the academic community [15, 16] is assessing how much the child or young person actually does understand.

*Ethnicity*
- Studies may be global and the consent/assent process should always respect the local culture, religion and attitudes towards health care [17].
- The consent process may need adapting, e.g. in Asian or tribal African societies, because though the parent may be the legal guardian, the key decision maker may be a family elder or tribal leader. Consent forms may therefore need space for several signatures or other identification symbols indicating consent.
- Qualified, independent translators should be used to avoid the risk of potential misunderstandings or possible breaches of confidentiality.

*Lifestyle and Best Interests*
- Protocols that are too complicated or time consuming for busy parents to consent to will find recruitment very difficult.

- Informed consent process needs to reflect any lifestyle changes, e.g. to school/home/social life. It may not always be in the best interests of the child to assent.
- 'The best interests of the child should always prevail over science and society' [4, 18], for example a child should not be consented to a trial involving multiple blood sampling if they are needle phobic.

*Puberty*
- Consent and assent needs to respect developing autonomy and have respect for their personal confidentiality.
- Consent for pregnancy testing is a difficult area and information needs to be very carefully written, especially for Catholic countries.
- Consenting teenagers to practice contraception while needed to protect a potential fetus in a study are fraught with ethical difficulties as paediatricians do not have family planning expertise. It may jeopardise a good doctor/parent relationship if the investigator sends the teenager to the family planning clinic without the parent's knowledge. Whilst legal for 'emancipated minors' in some countries, e.g. UK and USA, it may not be ethical.

*Cognitive and Fine Motor Development*
- This is important in the consent process as this may be impaired by disease, e.g., children in epilepsy trials will need simpler information sheets than normally required for their age due to possible IQ loss subsequent to fitting or somnolent effects of medication.
- Fine motor development is also important in the consent process as children are often proud to sign their names on an assent form – but may not be able to hold a pen properly if they are used to pencils. Also the signature varies from day to day so cannot be used as an audit tool.

*Level of Parental Supervision*
- This is fundamental to the success of a paediatric trial yet is rarely discussed in the literature. The family may be willing to consent/ assent but a stressful lifestyle may prevent compliance. Only investigators experienced with children and know their families well should be selected.

## Paediatric Clinical Trial Management in Relation to Consent/Assent

- Please refer to CESP guidelines for study site guidance [17].
- Use of child-specific SOPs should be considered for the fully informed consent/assent process.
- If the practical implications of the research have not been thought through, investigators may be presented with final unworkable protocols, which make consent and assent more difficult than it needs to be. (See chapter *'Study and Protocol Design for Paediatric Patients of Different Ages'*, this book.)
- Experienced paediatric investigators will only select projects they think they are likely to be able to consent/assent children for. Partly so they don't waste everyone's time and partly because they do not want to jeopardise a good doctor/patient relationship if the study has little chance of success.
- Paediatricians will also not take families through a lengthy consent/assent process if the research is not in the best interests of the child.
- ICH/E 11 [19] suggests that companies only use investigators who have paediatric experience. Physicians who treat a wide age range may have general experience with children but not specialist skills required to conduct studies in children. Consenting children by them would be inappropriate.
- The site should be checked to ensure there is adequate private space for the family to discuss the trial before and during the consent/assent process [20].
- The practice of competitive recruitment between sites, employed by some companies – should be avoided as this could unduly tempt the Investigator to pressurise the parents to consent their children.
- The consent and therefore the recruitment process will take much longer than adult trials. It is a good idea to promote paediatric trial training within the company so that colleagues from different departments are aware of the clinical trial needs.
- There is also a need to understand that paediatric trial metrics such as 'first patient in' will take longer partly because the consent process is more complicated than for adult studies. The budget will be higher and timelines longer.

## Information Sheets

Poorly prepared information sheets and assent forms may delay Ethics Committee approval and lead to recruitment failure. For fully informed consent and assent in parents and children the Information Sheets need to:

- Contain information required for informed consent (purpose, risks, possible benefits, requirements, procedures, alternatives, data protection, etc.) in language that is easy to understand.
- Be as short as possible by avoiding repetition and be as concise and clear as possible.
- Summaries of information can be in a non-scientific tabular form.
- The location of an investigator site and the ethnicity of the surrounding population may determine an increased demand for interpreters. Consent and assent will be severely limited if information sheets are not translated into the prevailing second language.
- Be in a language and form that parents and children communicate in best. Populations with limited education may not be able to read even the translated version. Audio or pictorial information in this instance is essential.
- *Avoid jargon!* Some children think that 'study' is what they do for their teacher; a 'trial' is something to do with being bad and may think that 'airways' are vapour trails in the sky.
- Remember that parents of sick babies or children are likely to be tired, stressed and not absorb information properly so information needs to be clear, honest but not frightening.

## Conclusions

Consent/assent is a challenging but essential element in paediatric trial management. Careful planning and a family-centred approach is needed to make sure child participation in a trial fully meets legal and ethical standards and that they are included in decision-making, commensurate with their development and legal status. With patience and good teamwork between company and investigator sites it can be done well. This will significantly increase the recruitment rate and compliance needed for successful paediatric trials and engender better medicines for children.

## References

1   Regulation of the European Parliament and of the Council on medicinal products for paediatric use and amending Council Regulation (EEC) No 1768/92, Directive 2001/83/EC and Regulation (EC) No 726/2004. Soon available in English at http://www.europarl.europa.eu/activities/expert.do?language=EN

2   Lamprill J: Paediatric trials: Balancing profit & ethical safeguards. Clin Res Focus 2005;16:13–18.

3   http://www.cdc.gov/nchstp/od/tuskegee/time.htm

4   http://www.nihtraining.com/ohsrsite/guidelines/nuremberg.html

5   Gillick V: West Norfolk & Wisbech Authority [1986] AC112, [1985] 3WLR830, [1985] 3All ER 402 HL.

6   European Parliament 'Directive 2001/20/EC of the European Parliament and the Council: on the approximation of the laws, regulations and administrative provisions of the Member States relating to the implementation of good clinical practice in the conduct of clinical trials on medicinal products for human use'. Available via http://europa.eu.int/eur-lex/pri/en/oj/dat/2001/l_121/l_12120010501en00340044.pdf

7   Royal College of Paediatrics and Child Health: Ethics Advisory Committee. Guidelines for the Ethical Conduct of Medical Research Involving Children. Arch Dis Child 2000;82:177–182.

8   Wendler DS: Assent in paediatric research: theoretical and practical considerations. J Med Ethics 2006;32:229–234.

9   Johnson KM, Colburn P, Hudson S, Venneman M, Kearns G: Children in research speak for themselves. Clin Pharm Ther 1999;65:176.

10  Smalley A: Needle phobia. Paediatrc Nurs 1999:11:17–20.

11  Informed Consent for Trial Subjects: ICH Harmonised Tripartite Guidelines for Good Clinical Practice 4.8.7. Marlow, Institute of Clinical Research, p 25.

12  Alderson P: Ethics, the rights of the child, and legal considerations in paediatric clinical research. European Forum for Good Clinical Practice News, 2002, pp 10–12.

13  Alderson P, Montgomery J: What about me? Are children competent to decide on their own treatment, regardless of what their parents think? Health Service J 1996:22–24.

14  British Medical Association: Consent, Rights and Choices in Health Care for Children and Young People. London, BMJ Books, 2001, pp 4, 14, 16, 94.

15  Mackintosh DR, Molloy VJ: Opportunities to improve informed consent: frequently observed problems in processes and content. Appl Clin Trials 2003:42–48.

16  McNally T, Grigg J: Parents' understanding of a randomised double-blind controlled trial: how the results of a survey of parents of pre-school children involved in a trial of treatment for viral wheeze led to changes in research practice. Paediatr Nurs 2001;13: 11–14.

17  Guidelines for informed consent in biomedical research involving paediatric populations as research participants Ethics Working Group of the Confederation of European Specialists in Paediatrics (CESP). Eur J Pediatr 2003;162:455–458.

18  World Medical Association Declaration of Helsinki: Ethical Principles for Medical Research Involving Human Subjects. http://www.wma.net/e/policy/b3.htm

19  European Agency for Evaluation of Medicinal products ICH Topic E11: Clinical investigation of medicinal products in the paediatric population. CPMP/ICH/2711/99, London, 2000.

20  Moench E: The Challenges of Recruiting for Children with Depression. Business Briefing. Iselin, Pharmatech, 2003, pp 1–2.

Rose K, van den Anker JN (eds): Guide to Paediatric Clinical Research.
Basel, Karger, 2007, pp 59–64

..........................

# Collecting Blood and Tissue Samples in Paediatric Clinical Trials

*Sabine Fürst-Recktenwald*[a]    *Marianne Soergel*[b]

[a]Sanofi-Aventis Deutschland, GmbH, Frankfurt am Main, Germany;
[b]Novartis Pharma AG, Basel, Switzerland

## Introduction

Blood sampling is a key concern for many children asked to participate in a clinical trial, and for their parents. While Ethic Boards [1] tend to focus on the volumes to be collected, the discomfort and fears generated in the paediatric study participant may depend much more on other aspects:

- Is the professional who will take the sample skilled and experienced?
- How many attempts of sampling will be made if the first one is unsuccessful?
- Will they insist on a second attempt if they collected less than the desired amount?
- Will I/my parents be allowed to influence the procedure (e.g. contribute to the choice of the sampling site and of timing; decide upon the use of local anaesthetics; parental presence)?
- Will they force me if I change my mind and do not agree to be sampled? Will they be angry with me?

Obviously, these aspects depend to a large extent on the choice of the appropriate study sites. The answers to these questions should also be spelled out in the study protocol and in the patient's information for informed consent. This will encourage their inclusion as an integral part into the protocol discussion and related site instructions. It will also improve the families' or patient's position for insisting on an ethical approach to the thorny sampling issues of clinical studies.

## Blood Sampling

Collection of blood samples from children must take into consideration the age, weight and health of the subjects, the collection procedure, the amount of blood to be collected, and the frequency with which it will be collected. Whenever possible, blood should be taken from children at the same time that a clinically needed blood draw is performed to avoid 'extra' sampling procedures.

Blood samples can be obtained by direct venipuncture or through the use of intravascular catheters. Placing intravascular catheters should be considered for multiple blood samples.

Existing peripheral or central venous (or arterial) catheters should be used where present, as long as the study drug will be delivered through a separate infusion. It is crucial not to use the same catheters for infusion of the study drug and consequent blood draws for kinetic purposes.

The number of sampling attempts that will be acceptable should be limited to 2 or 3 in the study protocol and site instructions in order to avoid major discomfort caused by overzealous study nurses.

Local anaesthetic cream (e.g. EMLA) should be offered, as per patient's preference. Application of the cream needs to be performed at the appropriate time indicated for the specific cream used. Two sampling sites may be prepared in case of an unsuccessful first attempt.

It is highly recommended to fix the order in which the tubes should be filled if there's more than one and to generate a 'priority list' for the labs in case less than the minimal amount has been collected.

*Special Challenges in Different Age Groups*
*Newborns.* High haematocrit, slow blood flow, vacuum systems cannot be used. Clotting in the puncture cannula after 0.5–2 ml has been drawn is a frequent occurrence. Peripheral venous lines or ultrathin central venous lines don't work for sampling and may clot. Arterial lines work best, and should be used when in place for clinical purposes. Due to the high haematocrit, the amount of plasma or serum that can be gathered from a given sample volume will be lower than in older children.

*Infants and Toddlers.* Subcutaneous tissue being usually well developed, veins may be very challenging to find. 'Blind' puncture based on palpation and/or knowledge of 'fixed' superficial veins only may be necessary.

*Prepubertal Children.* Some have panicky, irrational fear of being sampled which they cannot overcome and which may be a reason to discontinue study participation.

*How Much?*

There's no internationally accepted guidelines about acceptable blood volumes which may be drawn from paediatric study participants. Some Institutions have issued their own guidelines. The one shown in table 1 is from the University of Pittsburgh.

Patients in very unstable cardiopulmonary condition may not tolerate a 2.5-ml/kg body weight (BW) sampling well. A sample volume of up to 1 ml/kg BW will be acceptable for every patient.

In studies in older children (e.g. not neonates, toddlers), where the direct benefit far outweighs this volume restriction and more blood is required and justified by the potential benefits, up to 9 ml venous blood/kg BW/8-week period may be considered with the latter figure being the absolute upper limit.

For patients who need regular blood transfusions for their clinical condition (e.g. oncology/haematology patients; premature babies), higher sampling volumes may be acceptable when sampling is timed shortly before a transfusion. Increasing the volume of transfusion correspondingly does not increase the risk for the patient as long as no additional donor is needed.

Both volume and frequency of blood sampling can be minimized by using micro-volume drug assays and sparse-sampling techniques, respectively [2, see also chapter by Pons and van den Anker, page 108 ff.]. This is especially relevant when studying very young children, premature babies and newborns.

The amount of blood requested must be carefully considered and discussed with the laboratory, and appropriate small tubes must be used, e.g. paediatric citrate tubes allow determination of all standard coagulation parameters with 1.3 ml of blood (to be exactly filled).

Using micro-sampling techniques, i.e. equipment designed to use the least amount of blood necessary for each test, is mandatory.

*Table 1.* Maximum allowable blood draw volumes (University of Pittsburgh Institutional Review Board)

| Body weight kg | Body weight lb | Total blood volume, ml | Maximum drawn in one blood draw (2.5% of total blood volume) | Maximum drawn in a 30-day period (5% of total blood volume) |
|---|---|---|---|---|
| 1 | 2.2 | 100 | 2.5 | 5 |
| 2 | 4.4 | 200 | 5 | 10 |
| 3 | 3.3 | 240 | 6 | 12 |
| 4 | 8.8 | 320 | 8 | 16 |
| 5 | 11 | 400 | 10 | 20 |
| 6 | 13.2 | 480 | 12 | 24 |
| 7 | 15.4 | 560 | 14 | 28 |
| 8 | 17.6 | 640 | 16 | 32 |
| 9 | 19.8 | 720 | 18 | 36 |
| 10 | 22 | 800 | 20 | 40 |
| 11–15 | 24–33 | 880–1,200 | 22–30 | 44–60 |
| 16–20 | 35–44 | 1,280–1,600 | 32–40 | 64–80 |
| 21–25 | 46–55 | 1,680–2,000 | 42–50 | 64–100 |
| 26–30 | 57–66 | 2,080–2,400 | 52–60 | 104–120 |
| 31–35 | 68–77 | 2,480–2,800 | 62–70 | 124–140 |
| 36–40 | 79–88 | 2,880–3,200 | 72–80 | 144–160 |
| 41–45 | 90–99 | 3,280–3,600 | 82–90 | 164–180 |
| 46–50 | 101–110 | 3,680–4,000 | 92–100 | 184–200 |
| 51–55 | 112–121 | 4,080–4,400 | 102–110 | 204–220 |
| 56–60 | 123–132 | 4,480–4,800 | 112–120 | 224–240 |
| 61–65 | 134–143 | 4,880–5,200 | 122–130 | 244–260 |
| 66–70 | 145–154 | 5,280–5,600 | 132–140 | 264–280 |
| 71–75 | 156–165 | 5,680–6,000 | 142–150 | 284–300 |
| 76–80 | 167–176 | 6,080–6,400 | 152–160 | 304–360 |
| 81–85 | 178–187 | 6,480–6,800 | 162–170 | 324–340 |
| 86–90 | 189–198 | 6,880–7,200 | 172–180 | 344–360 |
| 91–95 | 200–209 | 7,280–7,600 | 182–190 | 364–380 |
| 96–100 | 211–220 | 7,680–8,000 | 192–200 | 384–400 |

Adapted by Rhona Jack, PhD, August 2001; Children's Hospital and Regional Medical Center Laboratory, Seattle, Wash., USA. This information is similar to that used by the Committee on Clinical Investigations at Children's Hospital in Los Angeles, and at Baylor College of Medicine in Dallas, Tex., USA.

*Consent/Assent*

School-age children (lower age limit 5–7 according to local rules), must assent verbally to blood draws for research purposes and this should be documented in research and clinical records.

Adolescents (from age 12–14 years) may co-sign the parental consent form if desired by the investigator or parent.

All minors (anyone under 18) must have a parent or guardian sign a consent form giving permission to draw blood from their child for research purposes.

## Tissue Sampling

Tissue sampling might occasionally be applicable in paediatric clinical trials, e.g. with liver or kidney biopsies, bone marrow aspiration, collection of fluids such as cerebral spinal fluid (CSF) or bronchial fluids, or sampling within endoscopic examinations. All these are invasive procedures that should only be used when clinically necessary and not outside standard medical care. For most of these procedures sedation will be required (especially in young children) and safe sedation of children undergoing diagnostic and therapeutic procedures has to be ensured.

Non-invasive sampling procedures, such as urine and saliva collection, may suffice if the correlation with blood and/or plasma levels has been documented [see also chapter by Pons and van den Anker, this book]. Examples include theophylline therapy in asthmatic children where both saliva and urine can be used with high reliability as alternative biological fluid in pharmacokinetic research. Saliva may be used as a non-invasive method of measuring gentamicin serum concentrations to guide dosage adjustments in patients with good correlation when the drug was administered once-daily [2–4].

## References

1 Royal College of Paediatrics and Child Health: Guidelines for the ethical conduct of medical research involving children. Arch Dis Child 2000;82:177–182.
2 FDA, CDER, CBER, Draft Guidance for Industry: General Considerations for Pediatric Pharmacokinetic Studies for Drugs and Biological Products. November 1998.
3 Brown RD, Campoli-Richards D: Antimicrobial therapy in neonates, infants and children (review). Clin Pharmacokinet 1989;17(suppl 1):105–115.
4 Butler D, Kuhn R, Chandler M: Pharmacokinetics of anti-infective agents in paediatric patients (review). Clin Pharmacokinet 1994;26:374–395.

Rose K, van den Anker JN (eds): Guide to Paediatric Clinical Research.
Basel, Karger, 2007, pp 65–77

..........................

# Paediatric Formulations

*J. Breitkreutz*[a]   *C. Tuleu*[b]   *D. Solomonidou*[c]

[a]Institute of Pharmaceutics and Biopharmaceutics, Heinrich Heine
University Düsseldorf, Düsseldorf, Germany; [b]School of Pharmacy,
University of London, London, UK; [c]Novartis Pharma AG, Pharma
Development, Basel, Switzerland

When the necessity of better medicines for children is mentioned, most people think of the development of new substances. The majority of people are comparatively unaware that in drug treatment in children there is an additional issue that adds significant complexity to drug development: small children cannot swallow tablets, and the best medicine is useless if it tastes so bad that the baby refuses to take it. Parents might succeed if the medicine has only to be given once, but not if the treatment has to be given for a longer period of time. Adequate formulations for children's medicines is a technical challenge that has been underestimated in the past. It is an area that needs more attention especially as the registration authorities of the USA and the EU are now increasingly asking for marketable paediatric formulations as a condition of paediatric incentives or even for the entire registration.

## Introduction

An appropriate drug formulation is the basis of an efficient drug therapy in children and it should allow administering medicines accurately and safely. If children refuse the intake of the medicine or if the formulation concept fails due to a paediatric particularity, the efficacy of the therapy is at risk and medication errors are probable. However, the paediatric population represents a vulnerable group and comprises a wide range of developmental levels, physiological particularities and age-related abilities. Moreover, therapeutic outcomes can be even further complicated by the fact that a third contributor (parents, caregivers, nurses) is also involved.

The pharmaceutical companies are not always able to provide a formulation for a single drug substance, comprising all ages, development stages and specificities of children's health state mainly due to the unfavourable physicochemical properties of the compound itself. In addition, there is only limited knowledge available on the acceptability of different dosage forms, administration volumes, dosage form size, taste and, importantly, the acceptability and safety of formulation excipients in relation to the age and development status of the child.

As a consequence, the development of the best-suitable drug products for children is a major challenge in industrial drug development. The same issue has to be carefully reflected in sponsor-independent clinical research as inappropriate drug formulations may significantly influence the outcome of the study.

One of the most important issues in the development of medicines for children is the most appropriate dosage form in relation to age. Few studies have been performed to survey the use of different formulations in children. In particular, there are concerns about the age at which young children can safely swallow conventional tablets and capsules. Whilst this has not often been examined directly in the literature, there is indirect evidence from an examination of prescriptions for different dosage forms in relation to age and anecdotal reports of very young children being trained to manage oral solid dosage forms for chronic illness such as leukaemia and HIV. Suppositories may be prescribed more commonly for children <5 years whilst the prescription of dosage forms such as inhalers and topical treatments remains relatively constant in relation to age through childhood.


## Drug Administration Routes

The oral route of administration is commonly used for dosing medicinal products to children and consequently many medicines should be available in both liquid and solid oral dosage forms. The variety of different oral dosage forms available such as solutions, syrups, suspensions, powders, granules, effervescent tablets, orodispersible tablets, chewable tablets, chewing gum, mini tablets, innovative granules, conventional immediate release and modified release tablets and capsules makes this route extremely useful for the administration of medicines to children of a wide age range.

*Peroral Liquid Formulations*

Liquid formulations include solutions, syrups, suspensions and emulsions and are most appropriate for younger children (e.g. birth to 8 years) who are unable to swallow capsules or tablets. The dose volume is a major consideration for the acceptability of a liquid formulation. Typical target dose volumes for paediatric liquid formulations are ≤5 ml for children under 5 years and ≤10 ml for children of 5 years and older. However, the more palatable the formulation, the higher the dose volume which will be tolerated. If taste and drug release characteristics are appropriate, solutions are preferred over suspensions due to better oral acceptance and dose uniformity. Furthermore, it is necessary for suspensions that sufficient information on the handling prior to administration is provided, i.e. need to shake the product to ensure correct dosing.

Devices for the delivery of liquid paediatric medicines should allow accurate dose measurement and simple, controlled administration. Household spoons should not be recommended as dose delivery devices for children's medicines. If a spoon is considered to be appropriate for dose delivery, a 5-ml spoon designed and manufactured to an appropriate international, EU or national standard should be provided by the manufacturer.

Validated measuring spoons and cups are convenient for toddlers and children who can use them without spilling but it is difficult to control administration if the child is uncooperative. They are commonly available in a total volume of 10 ml, with and without calibration lines for lower volume, i.e. 5 and 2.5 ml. Measuring spoons and cups can be used for all liquid preparations such as suspensions and solutions.

Graduated pipettes and oral syringes are particularly convenient for infants and young children who are not able to use either spoons or cups and allow accurate dose measurement and controlled administration to the buccal cavity for all ages. These dosing devices are recommended for medication with a narrow therapeutic window where accurate dosing is mandatory. Graduated pipettes intended for administration directly into the mouth must not be made of material that could break or cause damage.

Delivery of liquid medicines as a small volume measured as drops may be convenient, particularly for infants and young children. However, the accuracy of dosing depends on several factors, especially the angle at which the dropper bottle is held and the viscosity and density of the preparation.

The device selected should be appropriate to the volumes to be measured, therapeutic index of the active substance, type and taste of formulation and ease of administration in practice. Foaming after reconstitution or in use may affect accuracy of measurement and appropriate information and warnings should be given.

To avoid potential for error, graduations on dosing devices should only be stated in millilitres or fractions of a millilitre. If markings in other units can be justified (e.g. milligrams), the device must be labelled for use with that product only.

Design and labelling of the device should enhance use and should be evaluated by testing. Compatibility of all components of the device and labelling should be established, as should resistance to common washing procedures. Information should be provided to the user.

*Peroral Solid Formulations*

Classical solid drug formulations comprise granules, powders, capsules and tablets. Solid oral dosage forms such as tablets and capsules can offer advantages of greater stability, high content uniformity, and accuracy of dosing and improved portability over liquid formulations. Palatability is rarely an issue with film and/or sugar coats used to improve taste. The primary limitation for paediatric use is that solid oral dosage forms can present significant problems for young children and adolescents who have difficulty swallowing. The age at which children can swallow intact tablets or capsules is highly dependent on the individual and the training and support they receive from healthcare professionals and caregivers. It has recently been demonstrated that about a half of a group of preschool children may learn the swallowing of conventional tablets by special training programmes but modern solid drug preparations like multiple-unit drug carriers or rapidly dissolving formulations seem to be superior for most children.

Fast-dissolving drug formulations for administration into the buccal cavity are novel attractive dosage forms for paediatric use as they combine the major advantages of solid drug formulations, such as improved drug stability, with easy administration and swallowing. After placing fast-dissolving wafers or lyophilisates onto the tongue they dissolve within seconds and release the drug substance. The major limitation for this principle can potentially be the unpleasant taste.

Granules, powders and mini tablets are mostly designed for the extemporaneous preparation of a liquid or suspension by dissolving in water or mixing with food just before application. Attention should be drawn to the drug stability in the prepared liquid preparation as drugs can rapidly degrade when coming into contact with water and food ingredients. Effervescent or fast-dissolving tablets and chewable tablets may be considered as alternative dosage forms.

Multiple-unit preparations for paediatric use are built of small-sized pellets or mini tablets. Dose adaptation of multiple-unit systems is easy, comfortable, less risky and more exact than splitting tablets into pieces or crushing them to a powder. Modification of the release of the drug can be achieved for each unit, e.g. by film coating. The units are marketed in a multiple-dose container together with a suitable measuring device or as single doses contained in a capsule or tablet. As small-sized units can pass the pylorus in the fastened and full state of the stomach, they are able to minimize variations in bioavailablity and accelerate the onset of drug action. Mini tablets exhibit an excellent dose and shape uniformity.

Despite the advantages mentioned beforehand, oral drug formulations show some obstacles and drawbacks in paediatric use. General limitations include the lack of complete intestinal drug absorption, varying gastrointestinal transit time, and changing pH conditions along the gastrointestinal tract with the age of the paediatric population. Especially neonates and infants up to 1 year may have gastric fluid pH values of between 5 and 7 in the fasting state instead of the normal range of pH 1–2 as well as transit times of several days. Thus, cautious use of enteric-coated formulations is requested in these subpopulations.

*Buccal Formulations*
The buccal administration of drugs in children has gained an increased interest in the most recent time due to novel drug dosage forms

and more palatable drug formulations. However, one should be aware that the drug absorption after buccal administration is composed of transmucosal drug permeation within the mouth as well as intestinal absorption after swallowing the drug-containing saliva. Hence, the pharmacokinetic profiles of a drug can vary inter- as well as intraindividually. Fundamental limitations associated with this mode of administration are the lack of co-operation of children, their difficulties in coordination, and the risk of choking and aspiration. As anticipated, taste is one of the major determinants of mucosal contact time and of particular importance for products designed especially for children.

### Rectal Formulations

The rectal route of administration can be used to achieve either local (e.g. laxative, anti-inflammatory) or systemic (e.g. antipyretic, analgesic, anti-nauseant, anticonvulsive, sedative) effects.

In paediatric, as in adult therapy, rectal dosage forms may be indicated for a number of reasons:
- The patient cannot take medications orally or the oral route is contraindicated, for example due to nausea and vomiting.
- The oral dosage form is rejected because of palatability issues.
- Immediate systemic effects are required, for example to manage repetitive epileptic seizures.
- Local effects are required, for example laxative or anti-inflammatory preparations.

However, when administering rectal preparations to paediatric patients, there is a danger of the dosage forms being expelled prematurely. In addition, concordance and compliance may be lower than for oral dosage forms, as the rectal route of administration is poorly accepted by patients and caregivers in certain countries and cultures. Furthermore, the bioavailability of most drugs is very limited after rectal administration. The rectal absorption site shows a minor absorption area, a lack of active drug transporters and a very limited fluid volume for dissolving the drug. Therefore, important drug substances like levodopa, phenytoin or penicillins cannot be administered rectally.

### Nasal Formulations

Whereas nasal preparations like drops or ointments have been widely used for years for the local treatment, the nasal route provides direct access to the systemic circulation, and may be an attractive (needle-free) alternative to invasive administrations, especially in non-compliant patients and for peptide-like drugs. The use of preservatives in nasal multiple-dose containers that may be toxic for small children has meanwhile been resolved. Due to recent progress in packaging materials and development of novel drug delivery systems, the use of preservatives is no longer required.

*Injectable Formulations*

For neonates, infants, and seriously ill children the parenteral route of administration is still a perceivable alternative. The medication may be administered either intravenously, intramuscularly, or subcutaneously. Intramuscular injections are generally painful for children, so the intravenous route may be preferred if several regular injections are required. Many active substances for injection will be presented as lyophilised powders to be reconstituted before administration. Most doses for neonates, infants, and toddlers will require withdrawal of a dose volume which is less than the total volume after reconstitution. The facility to accurately measure small volumes of injections intended for newborns and young children is of particular importance. Concentrations of active substances should be such that the dosage volumes required can be measured with standard syringes and without further dilution. If dilution is required after measurement and prior to administration, it must be remembered that a significant extra quantity of active drug may be contained in the hub of the syringe, so appropriate instructions must be given. Failure to dilute very small volumes prior to intravenous administration or to flush them into the system may result in delays in delivering the drug or failure to deliver the whole quantity because of loss within administration apparatus.

The osmolarity of the preparation is a critical parameter. Hyperosmolar injections and extremes of pH may irritate small peripheral veins and produce thrombophlebitis and extravasation. Hypo-osmolar injections may induce haemolysis. The clinical need to reduce the fluid uptake, plasticizer desorption (e.g. phthalates) from and drug migration into the containers and catheters should also be thoroughly investigated as well as the punction pain or needle phobia of the child. Various needle-free injectors, spring-powered or gas driven, have been recently developed to overcome needle phobia. However, even administration with needle-free injectors may be painful. Additional obstacles are the more difficult handling, development and production costs by far higher than for common syringes and targeting the drug efficiently and safely into different tissues of the patients.

### Topical-Dermal and Transdermal Formulations

The transdermal route is restricted to a small number of appropriate active substances. In the paediatric population, the varying hydration status of the skin is a major problem that can affect drug permeation, e.g. the use of scopolamine transdermal patches had to be restricted to elderly children due to hallucinogenic reactions caused by unexpected elevated plasma concentrations. However, some dermal patches for local and systemic pain relief are successfully used.

### Inhalation Products

Inhalation is a suitable way to administer active substances to the lung. It is the preferred route of administration for patients with asthma. Other diseases such as infection in cystic fibrosis can also be treated locally by inhalation. In the future inhalation might become more important for the application of active substances for systemic treatment.

Advantages of the inhalation route over the oral route of administration include avoidance of hepatic first-pass metabolism. Inhalation might be an alternative route to parenteral application for systemic treatment, e.g. with peptides and proteins. Compared to the parenteral route, pain during application can be avoided.

The fraction delivered to the lung depends on several factors. One important factor is the ability of the patient to use the device correctly. Depending on their age children will have more or less difficulties with some of the devices. Problems with the coordination of the inhalation determine the effectiveness the drug reaching the lung. Furthermore, the low inspiration volume of paediatric patients often limits the proper use of drug-dosage forms for inhalation. Appropriate inhalational devices are rare, but electronic nebulizers, facemasks and spacers may improve the uniformity of the inhaled dose.

## Manipulation of Adult Dosage Forms

The manipulation of adult medicines for paediatric use should be the last resort, but at the same time it is recognised as an unavoidable and necessary operation in many cases in order to facilitate clinical investigations in paediatric populations or the treatment of children in an unlicensed or off-label manner. This section should be read in conjunction with the risks associated with the manipulation of adult medicines.

The following list of manipulations is not exhaustive, it serves chiefly to highlight practices of manipulating licensed products:

*Crushing Tablets*

The objective here is to reduce the monolithic tablet to a fine powder in which the active substance is assumed to be uniformly distributed, and which is amenable to dose reduction or to mixing in food or drink to facilitate ingestion. In the simplest situation a mortar and pestle might be used. A division of the powder might even be made by visual inspection in a domiciliary environment (obviously associated with a high risk of dosage error) or by weight, in proportion to the intended dose to be given. There is also the added risk of segregation of the active substance in the bulk powder caused by prolonged handling and vibration. In a hospital pharmacy environment, manipulations that may increase the homogeneity of the resulting 'bulk' powder might be as follows:

- Milling of the tablets in a small laboratory hammer mill. Changes in particle size may influence bioavailability. Temperature rises may increase the potential for chemical degradation or solid-state transitions, particularly in the case of steroids.
- An added manipulation frequently used in the hospital environment is the blending of powdered tablets with a lactose diluent, subsequently filled into powder sachets or hard gelatin capsules by hand or using a hand-filling machine to facilitate the preparation of batches of up to 100 or so. This manipulation requires technical skill in validation and operation.
- There is the danger that blending with lactose may be applied as a default operation when this is not relevant. For example, active substances which are primary amines (e.g. amlodipine) are more ap-

propriately formulated without lactose because of the well-known interaction and instability in the presence of such reducing sugars.

- There is also the risk that modified release tablets may be inadvertently crushed or manipulated in this way, so that their special advantageous properties are lost.

*Splitting Tablets into Segments*

From a practical point of view this seems a simple operation where the tablets are scored to facilitate such a manipulation. It relies on the assumption that the active substance will be uniformly distributed throughout the volume of the tablet. However, the potential for dosage error is more apparent with small tablets and low-dosage tablets (i.e. potent drugs where the active content may be in the sub-milligram range), and increases if the tablets are not scored even when using devices for containing and cutting tablets available and used in healthcare or domiciliary settings.

New tablet geometries like the Snap-Tab™ principle may improve the splitting of tablets and reveal more uniform segments than conventional tablets with a breaking notch.

Some tablets should not be manipulated in this way, for example, enteric-coated tablets, layered tablets (the matrix is not homogeneous) and many modified-release dosage forms; however, it may be possible to manipulate some matrix forms. There are some modern techniques like drug macrocrystals, drug embeddings in hydrocolloids or pellet-containing tablets that enable the splitting of monolithic preparations into pieces without compromising the principle of modified release.

*Opening Capsules*

This is a refinement on crushing tablets, in that the manufacturer has already established a powder matrix. As in the case of crushed tablets (see above), the capsule contents might be divided by visual inspection or weight with the attendant risks, or dispersed into drink/food to facilitate ingestion. Modified-release preparations of coated particles packed in capsules can usually be opened and dispersed into food or drink. The contents of the capsules may be manipulated into powder sachets or smaller capsules as above.

*Cutting Suppositories*

Again, this assumes a uniform distribution of the active substance in the suppository matrix. Accurate adjustment of dosage is difficult in this case, since very few suppositories are presented in a convenient shape facilitating halving by simple visual inspection. Cutting along a plane of symmetry (i.e. vertically rather than horizontally) would be an obvious solution and carries less risk of dosage error but the resulting shape may not be optimal for rectal insertion. Horizontal truncation of an asymmetric or bullet shape or rounded truncated cone carries the highest risk of dose error.

*Injectable Solutions Administered by Other Routes*

Using injections for oral administration is expensive, but in general this manipulation has the least potential for dosage error since many injections are dilute aqueous solutions, non-viscous, and a dosage reduction can be obtained if necessary with a small syringe, possibly after further dilution. Powders for injection (i.e. lyophilisates) may be taken up in a suitable diluent in the normal way prior to dose reduction.

For oral administration, an unpleasant taste could be a problem and will have to be considered unless nasogastric tubes are used. However, there are a number of more significant risks.

In the case of preserved or multidose injections these may contain benzyl alcohol, propylene glycol, or other substances, or have a pH or osmolality potentially harmful to neonates or children.

Also, the stability of injection solutions may be compromised on dilution, and in the absence of reliable technical information from the original manufacturer, it should not be assumed that the stability profile of the original product will be duplicated on dilution.

Injections have sometimes been given by the pulmonary route following nebulisation. Ignorance of the precise composition of the parent (adult) formulation could pose a significant safety risk in the case of injections stabilised with sulphite-based antioxidants which may provoke bronchoconstriction.

## Conclusion

The potential impact of the formulation of a medicine is often underestimated. A survey on recent clinical trials in children clearly demonstrated that despite the recommendation of the ICH Steering Committee on the use of appropriate formulations in paediatric drug trials, detailed information on drug formulation and administration was not adequately provided in highly-cited peer reviewed journals, even where the medicines were unlicensed and had to be manipulated before administration. It is unacceptable as the problems resulting from a lack of suitably designed medicines for children can include the child not taking the medicine, inaccurate dosing with increased risk of adverse reactions (over dosing), ineffective treatment (under dosing) and the use of extemporaneous formulations for children, which may exhibit poor or inconsistent bioavailability, low quality and safety. This can impair the reliability of the whole study, its validity and therefore the implementation of the treatment in clinical practice after complex, expensive and awaited clinical trials.

It is expected that now, with the appropriate attention and the speed of technical advances, strong progress in developing medicines adapted for children will take place over the coming years.

## References

1  Yeung WV, Wong IC: When do children convert from liquid antiretroviral to solid formulations? Pharm World Sci 2005;27:399–402.
2  Ansel HC, Allen LV, Popovitch NG: Pharmaceutical Dosage Forms and Drug Delivery Systems, ed 7. New York, McGraw-Hill, 1999.
3  Schirm E, Tobi H, de Vries TW, Choonara I, de Jong-van den Berg LTW: Lack of appropriate formulations of medicines for children in the community. Acta Paediatr 2003;92:1486–1489.
4  McElnay JC, Hughes CM: Drug Delivery – Buccal Route. E-EPT 2002;1:800–810.
5  Bunn G: Administration of oral liquids. Pharm J 1983;231:168–169.
6  Committee on Drugs: Inaccuracies in administering liquid medication. Pediatrics 1975;56:327–328.
7  Litovitz T: Implication of dispensing cups in dosing errors and pediatric poisonings: a report from the American Association of Poison Control Centers. Ann Pharmacother 1992;26:917–918.
8  McKenzie M: Administration of oral medications to infants and young children. US Pharm 1981;June/July:55–65.
9  Deeks T, Nash S: Accuracy of oral liquid syringes. Pharm J 1983;231:462.

10    Monk PM, Ball PA: The accuracy of a paediatric dosing device. Aust J Hosp Pharm 1999;27:323–324.

11    Pugh J, Pugh CH: Accuracy of measurement of 2.5 ml dose by oral syringe and spoon. Pharm J 1994;253:168–169.

12    Reis EC, Roth EK, Syphan JL, Tarbell SE, Holbkov R: Effective pain reduction for multiple immunization injections in young infants. Arch Pediatr Adolesc Med 2003;157: 1115–1120.

13    Reis EC, Holubkov R: Vapocoolant spray is equally effective as EMLA cream in reducing immunization pain in school-age children. Pediatrics 1997;100:E5.

14    Cassidy KL, Reid GJ, McGrath PJ, Smith DJ, Brown TL, Finley GA: A randomised double-blind, placebo-controlled trial of the EMLA patch for the reduction of pain associated with intramuscular injection in four- to six-year-old children. Acta Paediatr 2001;90:1329–1336.

15    Phelps SJ, Helms RA: Risk factors affecting infiltration of peripheral venous lines in infants. J Pediatr 1987;111:384–389.

16    Phelps SJ (ed): Teddy Bear Book, Pediatric Injectable Drugs, ed 6. Bethesda, American Society of Health-Systems Pharmacists, 2002.

17    Anonymous: Paediatric Injectable Therapy Guidelines. Liverpool, Royal Liverpool Children's NHS Trust, 2000.

18    Standing JF, Khaki ZF, Wong IC: Poor formulation information in published pediatric drug trials. Pediatrics 2005;116:e559–e562.

Rose K, van den Anker JN (eds): Guide to Paediatric Clinical Research.
Basel, Karger, 2007, pp 78–86

......................

# Central Laboratory in Paediatric Clinical Trials

*Marietta M. Henry*

Covance Central Laboratory Services, Indianapolis, Ind., USA

## Introduction

Twenty years ago only a few paediatric clinical trials were being carried out. Safety labs (chemistry panel, complete blood count [CBC], urinalysis) were often the only tests performed. The number of paediatric clinical trials has increased rapidly since 1997 because the FDA and the EMEA became interested in the paediatric safety and efficacy of pharmaceutical drugs. As a consequence, the numbers of tests requested for paediatric clinical trials have increased exponentially.

## Evolvement of Central Laboratories

Central laboratories have evolved over the last decades in line with clinical trials becoming increasingly international. They have evolved into a service that has the ability to instruct investigator sites, provide visit-specific kits for the standardised collection, process laboratory specimens, interact with the investigator site to provide clean demographics for the laboratory data, manage transport of specimens to the laboratory and provide an electronic data reporting system. With the increasing number of paediatric trials that have to meet the standards applied to adult trials, central laboratories offer all the aforementioned services plus they work with pharmaceutical companies and clinical investigators to decrease blood volumes, offer paediatric reference ranges and share their knowledge with investigators and trial sponsors.

Esoteric testing is now routine in paediatric clinical trials. The exploration of bone health in children is taking place in multiple clinical studies – in children with asthma who use inhaled glucocorticoids, in HIV-positive children, in children with anorexia, in studies on depression, attention-deficit hyperactivity disorder and bipolar disorders. The tests required for trials using humanized monoclonal antibodies in the treatment of juvenile rheumatoid arthritis not only include rheumatoid factor but also a number of cytokines and other markers of inflammation. The push to understand and treat paediatric type II diabetes involves testing for multiple inflammatory markers, lipids, cytokines, EKGs and sex hormones as well as haemoglobin A1C and plasma glucose levels.

All of this testing cannot be performed on a minimum of 8 ml of blood or some other small amount. Many of the esoteric tests are not 'child friendly', requiring more serum or plasma than a whole panel of chemistry tests. There is frequently a need for repeat testing in order to deliver a result. The tests themselves are not automated and may be less than robust in terms of performance. And most of the research-use-only tests that are being investigated as biomarkers have neither paediatric reference ranges nor publications in the literature to provide any guidance about what is normal in a child.

Reference ranges for the esoteric analytes sometimes will be based on Tanner stages of development. This will often require that an attachment in the protocol defines Tanner stages in order that good documentation will be provided by the investigator site. Non-paediatricians and clinical research associates may need to be reminded about the effects of puberty on analytes such as sex hormones and leptin.

Often a pharmaceutical company wants to use the same amount of testing as used in an adult clinical trial. But the blood loss will not be acceptable to the investigator site or the Institutional Review Board. The pharmaceutical company should consult with the central laboratory in order to plan a safe combination of testing using the least amount of blood. Calling the laboratory to find out the absolute minimum amount of blood required may lead to efficiencies of use of the serum/plasma at the central laboratory. The investigator site must then understand and partner with the pharmaceutical company to draw the full amount of blood requested or some testing may not be performed. Central laboratories for clinical trials should be able to prioritize testing on minimum amounts of blood by protocol visit, if necessary.

## Advantages of Central Laboratories

Central laboratories work only with clinical trials specimens. They provide the same analytical method for an analyte through the length of a clinical trial with the same reference ranges. If a reagent vendor changes formulations or discontinues a reagent, the central laboratory will work to develop a correlation formula for the new formulation. Central laboratories also provide favourable transportation rates and efficiencies of auditing for pharmaceutical companies – only 1–4 global laboratory sites in contrast to multiple local laboratories, several large general referral laboratories and academic laboratories.

## Basic Rules for Paediatric Clinical Trials

Paediatric clinical trials are less frequent than adult trials. When preparing a trial, the responsible person needs to be aware that answers given to him by a technician in the central laboratory may apply mainly to adults. Children are vulnerable and deserve a reduction of potential errors from the beginning. Always ask for the most senior person available when a trial involves children.

### Blood Collection Tubes

One of the challenges of paediatric clinical trials is that the size of the blood collection tube may be non-standard due to the need to collect minimum amounts of blood. The investigator site does not easily handle tiny tubes and the non-standard sizes require special adaptors for centrifuge cups. The advent of the 'partial draw' blood collection tubes and other types of tubes that allow drawing of minimum volumes with a larger tube helped. However, in a paediatric clinical trial where multiple analytes must be measured and allowable blood volumes are restricted, one often still may use very small tubes. When minimum blood volumes are calculated, the investigator must understand that providing less than the requested volume of sample may mean that not all tests are reported.

### Blood Collection Methods
*Finger Stick or Heel Stick.* Collecting blood by finger stick or heel stick is *never* recommended in paediatric clinical trials. If you do decide to allow heel sticks for infants under 2 months, the sites need to be reminded of the potential for haemolysis if:

- Residual alcohol is on the skin puncture site. Alcohol lyses red blood cells. Ensure the site is dry prior to puncture.
- Excessive squeezing is used. Squeezing will cause haemolysis. It is better to perform a second skin puncture. Never re-stick the same site or re-use a lancet.
- The collection tube is scraped against the skin. This will often mechanically lyse the red blood cells. The drops of blood should fill the collection tube by capillary action.
- Shaking of the micro-collection tube is too vigorous.

Heel stick or finger stick specimens will have a different glucose result than venipuncture due to the amount of arterial blood present in the mix of venous and arterial blood in the capillaries. However, one may also see significant differences in the calcium, total protein and potassium in capillary blood. Except for glucose, the other analytes mentioned are lower in capillary blood than in venous blood [1]. Mixing finger sticks and venipunctures is not recommended.

### Paediatric Venipuncture
Venipuncture is more effective and less painful than heel sticks with manual lancets [2]. A central laboratory may provide either vacuum tubes for blood collection with needle sizes appropriate for the size of a patient or may provide butterfly needles and tubing. Intravenous catheters for multiple timed draws (heparin locks) may also be provided. Although a butterfly needle and tubing is often requested by investigators, slow flow of blood through the tubing may lead to microclotting of platelets or clotting of an anticoagulated specimen. In general, central laboratories prefer a needle and vacuum tube due to fewer cancellations for clotting or haemolysis. However, vacuum systems do not work in small children due to the size of their veins. EMLA cream cannot be dis-

tributed globally from a central laboratory due to prescribing regulations.

### Reasons for Cancellation of Paediatric Specimens

*Haemolysis*
The most common reason for cancellation of laboratory tests is haemolysis. Haemolysis is a function of the phlebotomy technique or the processing of the blood after collection.

*Processing*
Most haemolysis issues occur in the processing of the specimens. If the blood is not allowed to clot well (usually 30 min after collection), there is an increased chance of red blood cells being present in the serum/plasma. If blood is left on the clot or a gel for greater than 30 min, there is a risk of an elevated potassium (due to breakdown of red blood cells) and a lowered glucose (due to metabolism by cells). Some small protein analytes may be attacked by serum/plasma proteases and a falsely low level is seen when the serum/plasma is left on the clot too long.

A centrifuge must be used that can achieve a speed of at least 1,500 $g$ (preferably 2,500 $g$) for 15 min. The centrifuge should receive documented maintenance checks, be placed on a level surface and should run smoothly. The person using the centrifuge must understand the concept of balanced loading. The brake on the centrifuge should *never* be used to stop the spinning since a sudden stop may cause red blood cells to be thrown up into the serum/plasma layer. The blood should never be poured from the collection tube after centrifugation but should be carefully removed with a disposable pipette, avoiding the gel layer and the plasma/platelet/WBC interface (table 1).

Serum or plasma with no visible red blood cells or haemolysis at the investigator site may have sufficient haemolysis from red blood cells that certain chemistry tests or coagulation tests are cancelled.

*Clotting*
The second most common reason for cancellation of specimens is clotting of the CBC specimens. This is due to both phlebotomy and patient reasons:

**Table 1.** Recommendations for a centrifuge used in clinical trials

| |
|---|
| The centrifuge must be able to reach a speed of 1,500 *g* for no less than 15 min at 22°C |
| The centrifuge must have a lockable lid |
| The centrifuge must include special bio-containment vessels, e.g. sealed rotors or safety cups |
| The centrifuge should not be equipped with a manual brake |
| The centrifuge must have a swing-out bucket rotor to minimize re-mixing of the serum/plasma with red blood cells, white blood cells and platelets |

*Phlebotomy-related reasons for clotting of anticoagulated whole blood:*
- A difficult draw, necessitating movement of the needle in the soft tissue, with tissue fluid accumulating in the needle. This tissue fluid, with a high concentration of clotting factors, is then washed into the blood collection tube and clots or fibrin strands and microclots form prior to contact with the EDTA anticoagulant.
- Inadequate mixing of the anticoagulant with the blood. I recommend drawing the EDTA tube last and gently mixing it 4 or 5 times by inversion. It will help to have an assistant present to mix the blood after collection while the phlebotomist is caring for the child.
- Drawing the EDTA tube first instead of last when several blood collection tubes are required at a visit. Tissue fluid is allowed into the needle and flushed into the collection tube.

*Patient-related reasons for clotting of anticoagulated whole blood:*
- Patient has genetic predisposition to clotting quickly – deficiencies in protein C, protein S, factor V Leiden, etc.
- Tendency of some patients to develop microclots in the presence of EDTA. This appears to be an idiosyncratic response that may happen consistently in blood from a patient. It is more common in adults than in children.
- Presence of high concentrations of serum proteins, such as rheumatoid factor. This is postulated to make the platelets stickier, particularly at temperatures lower than body temperature. Certain diseases are associated with an increased occurrence of microclotting – rheu-

matoid arthritis, hepatitis C, multiple myeloma, AIDS, autoimmune diseases, sepsis/bacteraemia and infectious diseases. Platelets are part of the acute-phase defence in infectious diseases and children often have high platelet counts in the acute stages of an infectious disease.

- Leaving the tourniquet on too long with stasis of venous blood. The tourniquet should be placed for only 1 min. Blood collection should be promptly begun after the tourniquet is placed. Leaving the tourniquet on too long (over 1 min) can encourage clotting factors to activate (factor VII and von Willebrand factor).
- Placing the EDTA tube into the refrigerator prior to putting it in the transport kit may cause clotting or microclots. The EDTA tube is to remain at room temperature prior to and during transport. Putting the CBC blood into the refrigerator or exposing it to cold can assist in the generation of clots. Chilling to 4°C activates factor IV.
- Incorrect usage of a combination packaging kit (containing frozen specimens and ambient specimens).

**Packaging of Specimens**

It is important for the investigator site to properly package the specimens from a clinical trial. Central laboratories provide tested packaging that ensures that extremes of temperatures are avoided and special conditions (e.g. frozen specimens) are maintained. They can provide pictorial directions for packaging of infectious, non-infectious and combined modality shipments. They also can provide pre-printed airbills for the investigator site and dry ice in most countries. If the site incorrectly packages specimens, the courier company or import/export officials may turn the package back and the specimens will be out of stability, requiring a re-draw from the patient. The myriad of special paperwork required to bring specimens out of or into a country is well understood by central laboratories.

## Visit-Specific Kits

Part of a central laboratory's usefulness is the ability to provide visit-specific kits to the investigator site. The site's clinical coordinator only needs to open the correct visit box and all the supplies are present that are needed for specimen collection at that visit as well as the visit-specific requisition. The site performs what is required for that visit and only what is required. The coordinator does not have to hunt for specific tubes, needles or other supplies. All the tubes should have bar-code labels and the name of the testing is placed on the label of the transport vial in order to be sure that the correct specimen is sent to the central laboratory. Ease of use makes for fewer mistakes and fewer re-draws of specimens.

## Investigator Support

A central laboratory provides language-specific toll-free telephone lines for investigator sites in order to facilitate communication of alerts for abnormal laboratory results as well as for training or re-training if consistent errors are made. Kits may be ordered also. Common errors are well-known due to the volume of investigator sites serviced and proactive counselling is possible. When required, visits to an investigator site with poor performance can be arranged for one-to-one dialogue with the clinical trials coordinator.

## Conclusions

Central laboratories will become more and more routine in paediatric clinical trials as their standards approach the rigorous levels of adult testing. In all paediatric laboratory testing, it is important for both sides to pay extra attention to avoid waste of blood and other specimens. The search for biomarkers of diseases or response to drugs will continue in paediatric clinical trials as well as in adults. Current methods of testing for esoteric analytes require more blood than may be acceptable and often have no paediatric reference ranges.

## References

1 Blumenfeld TA, Hertelendy WG, Ford SH: Simultaneously obtained skin-puncture serum, skin-puncture plasma, and venous serum compared, and effects of warming the skin before puncture. Clin Chem 1977;23:1705–1710.
2 Larsson BA, Tannfeldt G, Lagercrantz H, Olsson GL: Venipuncture is more effective and less painful than heel lancing for blood tests in neonates. Pediatrics 1998;101: 882–886.

Rose K, van den Anker JN (eds): Guide to Paediatric Clinical Research.
Basel, Karger, 2007, pp 87–107

..................

# Study and Protocol Design for Paediatric Patients of Different Ages

*Oscar Della Pasqua*[a, b]   *Lothar-Bernd Zimmerhackl*[c]   *Klaus Rose*[d]

[a]Clinical Pharmacology & Discovery Medicine, GlaxoSmithKline,
Greenford, UK; [b]Leiden/Amsterdam Center for Drug Research, Leiden,
The Netherlands; [c]Department of Pediatrics I, Medical University
Innsbruck, Innsbruck, Austria; [d]Pediatrics, F. Hoffmann-La Roche Ltd.,
Pharmaceuticals Division, Basel, Switzerland

## Introduction

*Study Protocol and Protocol Rationale*

A clinical study protocol is a key document that forms the backbone of every single clinical trial. In principle, there are no differences between the contents of an adult and a paediatric protocol. It has to describe what is planned in the study, and why, when and how to achieve it. It has to include a high-level study rationale and list operational details. Due to the paediatric legislations in the USA and EU clinical research is now expanding from the adult population where the basics of clinical research are well established since decades to the paediatric population where most key players in clinical research are newcomers regarding their exposure to paediatric patients until now. A practicing paediatrician knows in depth the physiology and the mindset of a child. However, he will often be less knowledgeable in designing multi-centre international trial protocols. Vice versa, an industry scientist who is well experienced in writing study protocols for adults will have to learn a lot about children when he is assigned to write a clinical protocol for a paediatric indication. One of the reasons paediatric clinical research is more work intensive is that implementation of study protocols requires careful considerations regarding feasibility. Another hurdle is ethical committees, which have less experience with children and tend to block or at least slow the approval of paediatric trials as their exposure to paediatric research has been limited until now. Several specific challenges are covered in other chapters of this book, including how much blood volume and sample tissue can be asked for in a protocol, laboratory parameters, parental informed consent and assent to study participation by the child, appropriate paediatric formulations, and others.

The study rationale at the beginning of the protocol is key to making the trial possible. It should explain the objectives of the study in a language that can be understood by all members of an ethical committee, including those that are not medical doctors, PhD or PharmD by training. It should explain the key characteristics of the investigated drug in adults, compare the targeted disease(s) in adults and in children, give a high-level assessment of the therapeutic options available at present, and explain the expected therapeutic benefit as well as the expected scientific learning of the planned trial. As healthy children do not generally participate in clinical trials, the objective of every paediatric clinical study is always twofold. The included children have a health problem that is planned to be positively influenced by the study participation. Furthermore, scientific lessons are planned to be learned from the study participation. A balanced assessment of potential risks and benefits needs to be part of the study rationale. Failure to address these key issues in the study rationale will often result in additional questions from the ethical committee and/or in additional conditions that have to be met before the study can start. A good rationale will cost time in the beginning and will save time during study preparation and performance. It is also highly recommended to have any paediatric protocol reviewed by a paediatrician or a person otherwise competent in paediatric drug development.

*Study Planning*
Before operational details are planned, the study essentials should be discussed in the framework of the general clinical development plan with an appropriate expert. The following conditions need to be checked (fig. 1).

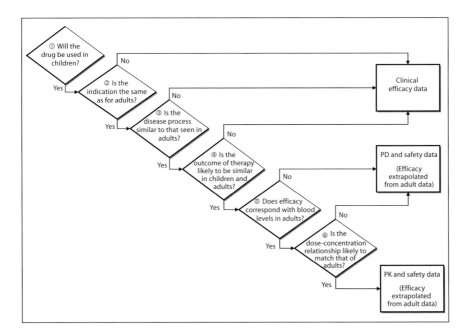

**Fig. 1.** Decision tree for the identification of clinical study requirements in a paediatric drug development program.

*Flow Sheet*

In the planning phase and in particular for the study period itself, the development of a flow sheet supports the surveillance and execution of the study.

## Study Population

ICH guideline ICH E 11 suggests 5 different age groups (table 1). Since this system defines only age as a descriptor of size and function, it disregards the evidence that multiple physiological processes develop beyond the proposed age boundaries, which determine, for example, homeostatic mechanisms and drug metabolism [1, 2]. Understanding how these factors change over time is essential for dose selection across the different phases of development [3]. Furthermore, in many in stances disease incidence and/or severity may be age-dependent, but not in agreement with the current ICH classification.

**Table 1.** ICH guideline ICH E 11

| ICH strata | Range |
|---|---|
| Pre-term neonate | <37 weeks gestation |
| Term neonate | 0–27 days |
| Infants and toddlers | 28 days to 23 months |
| Children | 2–11 years |
| Adolescent | 12–18 years |

The aforementioned developmental differences make the criteria for selecting the study population and dose rationale in a paediatric study slightly more complex than in adult studies. Population stratification must therefore be carefully considered in conjunction with aetiology and epidemiology aspects, instead of solely relying on ICH strata. On the other hand, patient selection will depend upon evidence for safety and tolerability across the different age groups. Whilst the dosage form is constant in an adult study, the availability of a suitable formulation will also play an important role in defining the study population.

*Healthy Subjects versus Patients*
Whilst healthy subjects are enrolled in most studies in early clinical development for adult indications, this option is generally not possible and ethically unacceptable for paediatric indications. The tenets of clinical research require that a subject should not be exposed to any unnecessary risks. Current guidelines also require that a subject be capable of consenting to participate in a trial, which infers capacity to understand the risks of the clinical research and his/her legal status to make independent decisions. These requirements often invalidate the use of healthy subjects in clinical paediatric research, which is in most cases performed in patients. A few exceptions exist in vaccine trials and when adolescents (>16 years of age) are legally granted adulthood status. However, even in such circumstances careful consideration of medical risk/benefit ratio is needed to decide on the enrolment of healthy subjects.

*Stratification versus Balanced Population*
Often supporting data on safety and epidemiology will impose staggering or stratification of the study population. The challenge is to iden-

tify a priori which factor or covariate best describes the developmental changes and hence which treatment arms or dose levels should be investigated. Common practice has been geared to stratification by age and/or weight. However, this approach disregards the role of other relevant physiological variables that may underlie the changes in function in the paediatric population.

In principle, it may be preferable to enrol groups of patients across a wide range of age, weight, or functional variable.

The need to stagger the clinical development across different age groups will be discussed later in conjunction with other safety aspects. It is important to realise that it will depend upon whether the necessary pre-clinical toxicology studies in animals have been performed and whether evidence is available for efficacy and safety in adults. These data will also be used as the basis for justification of the dosing rationale.

*Medical History and Disease Status*

Whilst it is commonly accepted that the development of a paediatric indication may be safer if progression is based on evaluation of older patients before exposing younger children to the investigational drug, this approach overlooks the aetiology of disease. Depending on the age of onset, disease status may be worse or severity of symptoms more pronounced in older age groups.

**Study Design**

*Development Phases*

Whilst most of clinical research has been based on sequential development, with rather well-defined stages and designs for the transition of a molecule from first-time-in-humans to a full pivotal efficacy trial, paediatric study protocols will have to cope with specific requirements of the paediatric patient population in that less strict separation between phases may be necessary and desirable. Such a requirement may impose the need for flexible or alternative study designs, which include considerations beyond the traditional, randomised, placebo-controlled study design. The ability to identify these differences is crucial to the success of a clinical study. Also, patient recruitment and overall incidence of disease in the target population ought to be taken into account when selecting study designs. Often the difficulties to recruit patients across a relevant range (based on age, weight or any other relevant physiological variable) are overlooked and become the cause of frequent protocol amendments.

*Early versus Late Clinical Development Studies*

As stated above, there is a less strict separation of the study phases when it comes to paediatric development, as one would not necessarily progress through clinical development by stand-alone studies aimed at single and multiple ascending dose escalation for pharmacokinetics, safety and tolerability, followed by a proof-of-concept, a phase IIb dose-ranging study followed by a pivotal efficacy trial.

Paediatric protocols must address relevant clinical development questions efficiently. It is not advisable to perform stand-alone studies. First, there will be feasibility and ethical hurdles in running a study which has a primary objective the characterisation of pharmacokinetics and safety and tolerability only. One must be aware of the patient's needs and find a compromise between scientific rigour to derive accurate information about pharmacokinetics, pharmacodynamics, safety and tolerability with the potential benefits of treatment in the target population.

The selection of any given study design should take into account the location and shape of the concentration-response curve. From a statistical point-of-view, clinical efficacy study designs can be categorised according to the classification proposed by Palmer [4]. Whilst most clinical study protocols in adults can be based on a randomised, double-blind, placebo-controlled, parallel group design with fixed sample sizes, such a protocol may turn out to be inappropriate or unethical in a paediatric indication.

These limitations may be overcome by the use of so-called data-dependent designs, which have been applied not only in exploratory research but also in confirmatory (regulatory) clinical studies. Data-dependent study designs were introduced progressively in clinical research in the early 1940s, and consist of sequential, group sequential, adaptive interim, response-adaptive and Bayesian adaptive designs.

## Minimal Detectable Difference

The minimal detectable difference is the smallest difference between the treatments or strength of association that one wishes to be able to detect. In clinical trials this is the smallest difference considered to be clinically important and biologically plausible. In a study of association, it is the smallest change in the dependent (outcome variable, response), per unit change in the independent (input variable, covariate) that is plausible.

## Parallel Design

A parallel-designed clinical trial compares the results of a treatment on two separate groups of patients. The sample size calculated for a parallel design can be used for any study where two groups are being compared.

## Crossover Study

A crossover study compares the results of a two-treatment regimen in the same group of patients. The sample size calculated for a crossover study can also be used for a study that compares the value of a variable after treatment with its value before treatment. The standard deviation of the outcome variable is expressed as either the *within-patient* standard deviation or the *standard deviation of the difference*. The former is the standard deviation of repeated observations in the same individual and the latter is the standard deviation of the difference between two measurements in the same individual.

## Study to Find an Association

A study to find an association determines if one variable, the dependent variable, is affected by another, the independent variable. For instance, a study to determine whether blood pressure is affected by salt intake.

## Success/Failure

The outcome of the study is a variable with two values, usually treatment success or treatment failure.

## 'Smart' Designs

Data-dependent designs offer alternatives to clinical research protocols that may be more efficient, i.e. giving a surer answer about the location and shape of the exposure-response curve, providing important data for subsequent regulatory studies. The objective of these designs is to increase the proportion of subjects allocated to effective treatment levels. In fact, these concepts can be widely applied in adult and paediatric protocols.

These include:

- enrichment approaches;
- titration design;
- the randomised withdrawal study.

### Enrichment Approaches

Prospective use of any patient characteristic – demographic, pathophysiologic, or genetic, and others – as inclusion criteria for selecting patients in a study is usually done to obtain a study population in which the drug effect is supposedly more likely to be detected. This practice, whilst not necessarily identified, goes on all the time. Enrichment designs can decrease heterogeneity, identifying a population capable of responding to the treatment and thereby increasing the rate of response, or increasing the number of events that will occur in the study. A higher number of responders to treatment increases statistical power. Enrichment can thus greatly facilitate 'proof-of-concept' studies. Implementation of enrichment design requires an interim evaluation of response, as defined by a biomarker or clinical endpoint. Non-responders are subsequently withdrawn from the trial or randomised to a different dose level or treatment. In paediatric protocols this approach warrants shorter duration of exposure of patients who do not respond to an ineffective treatment arm.

### Concentration-Controlled (Titration) Design

In traditional efficacy studies, patients are randomised to a dose level. However, this procedure ignores the role of individual pharmacokinetic factors, yielding drug exposures that do not cover the thorough concentration-response curve, i.e. one of the key objectives of early clinical development. The titration design eliminates this limitation, as it is based on the allocation of a patient to a concentration range, rather than a dose level [5]. Implementation of this design requires a monitoring phase under steady-state conditions to ensure compliance to randomisation levels. A placebo or complementary dose level is subsequently used to titrate the patient to the allocated concentration range. Requirements for monitoring of drug concentration and dose adjustment are based on sparse sampling of pharmacokinetics and simulation techniques. Details of the data analysis methodology will be discussed in another section (see *Data Analysis and Statistical Considerations*).

### Randomised Placebo-Withdrawal Design

In some circumstances, enrichment can be achieved by evaluating the drug effect by withdrawal of treatment in patients who have been identified as responders (fig. 2). This approach can be particularly useful to identify treatment outcome associated with symptomatic improvement [6].

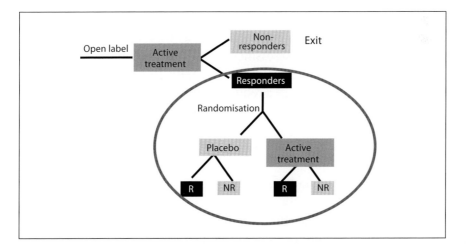

**Fig. 2.** Randomised placebo withdrawal study design. R = Responders; NR = non-responders.

From a practical point of view, randomised placebo-withdrawal studies offer every patient an opportunity to experience the potential benefits of active treatment. This results in better patient accrual in indications for which the use of a placebo arm may not be suitable or ethically acceptable (fig. 2).

A few points must be considered for the implementation of a randomised placebo withdrawal study, which may limit its application in early drug development. First, the use of parallel designs is often not possible due to varying disease features. Second, it cannot be used in testing drugs with a very long half-life (months) or drugs that induce irreversible changes. Third, it has limited value in unstable diseases and is not recommended for studying serious or life-threatening disease.


*Adapted Three-Stage Design*

In therapeutic indications such as rare diseases, accrual of patients becomes the main risk factor for the success of a clinical study. The concept of placebo withdrawal followed by re-randomisation of non-responders to a subsequent treatment level offers a very attractive alternative to standard designs. In a three-stage trial, all patients receive the active medication at a given stage of the trial, which consists of a sequence of three placebo-withdrawal stages (fig. 3). The main advantage of the approach is that non-responders are not excluded from the study, but are re-randomised to a different treatment level.

The formal statistical assessment of efficacy incorporates three separate stages, increasing the power of the study. In practice, the increase in statistical power results in a reduction in sample size of approximately 20–30%. The study design is, however, only applicable to chronic, stable conditions.


*Randomised Placebo Phase Design*

The randomised placebo phase design (RPPD) was used initially to assess the effect of monoclonal antibodies which produce permanent response or remission of disease. These treatments cannot be studied by placebo withdrawal or crossover designs. Design limitations are even

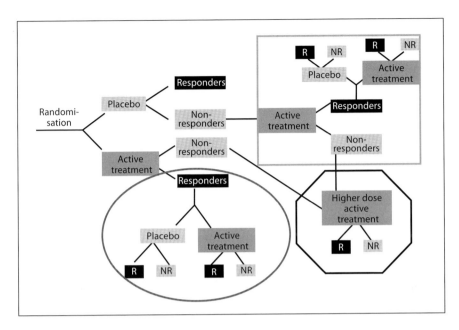

**Fig. 3.** Adapted three-stage design. R = Responders; NR = non-responders.

more important in the context of rare diseases or special population groups RPPD was develop to investigate disease-modifying therapies using survival endpoints.

Patients entering a RPPD study are not formally randomised to a placebo treatment arm, but to a randomised period during which placebo doses replace the active medication. The dependent variable is time from entry into the study to the time of a response (time to event). The independent variable is the time from entry into the study to the time of starting active treatment. The length of the placebo phase will predict the overall time to response if treatment is truly efficacious (fig. 4). Some subjects are censored if response occurs after termination of the study and dropouts may occur randomly or be related to treatment effect. The statistical significance of the treatment effect is based on a Cox proportional hazards regression (fig. 4).

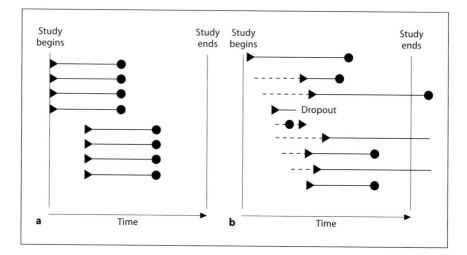

***Fig. 4.*** Randomised placebo phase design. ***a*** In standard clinical trials the duration of treatment with the active compound is fixed. The vertical bars represent the start and finish dates of the clinical trial. Each horizontal line represents one study subject. The triangles indicate the start of active treatment, whilst solid lines represent the treatment duration. Subjects are followed until they respond (closed circles). ***b*** Features of the randomized placebo-phase design (RPPD) trial. Subjects enter the trial at various times in the accrual phase. They are randomly assigned a period of time on placebo treatment (broken lines). At the randomly determined time, subjects blindly switch to active treatment (triangles). Subjects who do not respond during the trial (third, sixth and eighth subjects from top), and those who drop out (fourth subject from top) are censored. Some subjects may respond spontaneously while still on placebo (fifth subject from top). Adapted from Feldman et al. [7].

## Adaptive Designs

The use of enrichment approaches, concentration-controlled designs, placebo withdrawal and randomised placebo phase design presumes some knowledge and confidence about the location and shape of the concentration-response curve, as the allocated treatment levels are defined a priori, during the planning phase of the protocol. In many cases, however, there may not be enough understanding or confidence about the exact location and shape of the concentration-response curve. Therefore, performing studies with predefined, fixed doses or exposure levels may result in a higher development risk with potential failure to

**Table 2.** Rules for an adaptive design

| | |
|---|---|
| Allocation rule | how subjects will be allocated to available treatment arms |
| Sampling rule | how many subjects will be sampled at the next stage |
| Stopping rule | when to stop the trial (for efficacy, for harm, for futility) |
| Decision rule | interim decisions (to update the model, to change endpoint, to modify initial plan) |

**Table 3.** Opportunities and limitations of adaptive designs; adaptive designs enable adaptations to be real without losing credibility, transparency and rigour

| Opportunities | Limitations |
|---|---|
| Enhance design efficiency by learning as you go | Complex logistics for conducting the trial |
| Flexibility with respect to sample size | Need for short-term endpoints |
| Options for early stopping or/and change the initial design | Fast data capture and analysis required |
| Decrease costs associated with number of patients | More sophisticated statistical methodology |
| More accurate information with less resources | 'Accrual' and time bias. Knowledge of design can cause operational bias (later patients > probability of optimal treatment) |
| Additional breakpoints for checks of consistency | Population drift |

identify treatment effect in the target population. The possibility to make adjustments as one learns about the concentration-response curve may be very appealing in paediatric indications. Adaptive designs enable the implementation of adjustments in a formal manner, with statistical rigour and validity.

An adaptive design requires the trial to be conducted in several stages with access to the accumulated data. An adaptive design may have one or more rules (table 2).

At any stage, the data may be analysed and subsequent stages rede-signed taking into account all available data. During interim adaptation patient recruitment is not interrupted. A summary of the opportunities and limitations is presented in table 3. From a statistical point of view, the main differences between a standard randomised, double-blind, pla-cebo-controlled, parallel-treatment group and an adaptive design in-clude re-randomisation throughout the study and consequently an un-balanced distribution of patients across treatment arms. It also allows for variations in sampling schemes.

Not surprisingly, the ability to formally adapt a study results in sim-ilar logistics issues pertaining to traditional group-sequential designs, in particular, drug supplies. Adaptations should be performed by an inde-pendent third party with no conflict of interest, i.e. an Independent Data Monitoring Committee (IDMC) (table 3).

*Pharmacokinetic Studies*

As indicated previously, formal 'bridging' studies can be devised to explore dosing regimens associated with efficacious concentration levels. However, it is not recommended to set pharmacokinetics as the only objective in a paediatric clinical trial. It would not be easy to defend, ethically, a trial without any potential benefit to the child.

To overcome this limitation, it is advisable to combine pharmacoki-netic sampling with an open efficacy and tolerability study. The study is rolled out in two phases, each of which has a specific set of objectives.

Pharmacokinetics can be assessed after single dosing and at steady state in the same patient population. The main difficulty associated with paediatric studies is related to the requirement for frequent, serial blood sampling. This requirement derives from the use of non-compartmental pharmacokinetic analysis to derive information about drug exposure (AUC, area under the concentration-time curve) and other parameters, such as observed peak concentration ($C_{max}$) and the time associated with it ($T_{max}$). In fact, the same type of problem arises when serial sampling is required for efficacy and safety endpoints.

These limitations can be overcome by sparse sampling and limited population size in conjunction with a more sensitive data analysis meth-odology, which provides predicted population pharmacokinetic estimates instead of individual observed parameters. The population approach is a parametric statistical method, based on nonlinear regression techniques that yields population parameter distributions with estimates of a typical value for the population as well as providing a measure of inter-individual variability. Details of the population approach are provided under 'Data analysis and statistical considerations'.

## Endpoints

The primary variable ('target' variable, primary endpoint) should be the variable capable of providing the most clinically relevant and scientifically accepted evidence to support the primary objective of the trial. There should generally be only one primary variable and the one used when estimating the sample size. Pharmacokinetic parameters derived from drug exposure data, such as plasma concentrations, are also primary variables required to demonstrate safety, tolerability and efficacy.

In principle, the choice of the primary variable often relies on experience gained either in earlier studies or in the published literature, which shows whether or not a given variable is reliable and validated. This requirement, however, cannot be met in many paediatric indications due to the lack of experience with randomised clinical trials or clinical understanding of disease. The issue becomes evident in areas for which only subjective clinical scales or health outcome measures are available. It is not difficult to realise that many subjective questions may not be easily extrapolated to the context of a young child or an infant, who may not even be able to understand such questions properly. This situation imposes an open dialogue between investigators, clinical research scientists and regulatory agencies about the validity and acceptance of certain endpoints as proof of safety and efficacy for the purposes of a regulatory submission. Another important problem related to the validation of endpoints is the choice for alternatives where extrapolation is not possible. For instance, whilst $FEV_1$ is undoubtedly an ideal measure of efficacy for asthma, this endpoint is not reliably measurable in children under the age of 3.

In many cases, assessment of clinical outcome may not be straightforward and should be carefully defined. For example, it is inadequate to specify mortality as a primary endpoint without specifying whether proportions alive at fixed points in time or distributions of survival times over a specified interval will be compared. Similarly, when the endpoint is a recurring event, the measure of treatment effect may be defined in different ways, such as any occurrence during a specified interval, time to first occurrence, and rate of occurrence (events per time units of observation). The assessment of functional status over time in studying treatment for chronic disease presents other challenges in selection of the primary variable. There are many possible approaches, such as comparisons of the assessments done at the beginning and end of the interval of observation, comparisons of slopes calculated from all assessments throughout the interval, comparisons of the proportions of subjects exceeding or declining beyond a specified threshold, or comparisons based on methods for repeated measures data. Whatever the choice is, it is critical to specify in the protocol the precise definition of the primary variable as it will be used in the statistical analysis, including the clinical relevance and associated measurement procedures. These procedures may differ considerably from the adult population and should be highlighted in the protocol.

Secondary endpoints are either supportive measurements related to the primary objective or measurements of effects related to the secondary objectives. The correlation between primary and secondary endpoints in the paediatric population may not resemble findings in adults. Pre-definition and explanation of the relative importance and roles of secondary endpoints is essential for the interpretation of trial results. They are not important for the sample size calculation, but may influence the study design, the planning of patient visits, sample collection and statistical considerations.

### Dosing Rationale

*Evidence for Safety and Tolerability*
It is essential to consider whether the necessary pre-clinical toxicology studies in animals have been performed and whether evidence is available for efficacy and safety in adults. Depending on available evidence, staggering or stratification of the study population may be required (grouping by age, weight or any other relevant physiological variable).

*Concentration-Effect Relationships*

Dose selection for the paediatric indication must be based on pharmacokinetic-pharmacodynamic (PK/PD) relationships. Scaling factors for size must be treated as covariates. If the disease mechanisms and the clinical endpoint does not differ from the adult population, there will be many cases in which the concentration-effect relationship will be similar in both populations. In these circumstances bridging is the appropriate strategy for the clinical development of the paediatric indication. The rationale for dose selection should be such as to explore the exposure ranges that yield evidence of minimum and maximum clinical benefit.

If disease mechanisms are the same as in the adult population, but the endpoint is different or there is evidence for potential differences in PK/PD relationships, then doses should be evaluated that allow for exploration of the concentration-effect curve.

*Requirements for 'Bridging'*

The bridging strategy is applicable for indications for which evidence is available on the aetiology of disease and similarities in the concentration-effect relationship in the adult population. The principle underlying bridging studies are based on identifying a dosing regimen that produces drug levels in children that are equivalent to the exposure associated with efficacy in adults. Bridging approaches and adaptive designs can be implemented by modelling and simulation techniques. Such studies are cost-effective and have high informative value.

## Data Analysis and Statistical Considerations

Current practice in the design of studies for an indication in adults accommodates most statistical requirements by ensuring appropriate group size and frequent sampling. As previously described, the operational limitations associated with paediatric drug development impose careful consideration about data analysis prior to the start of the study. A particularly important issue is how to accurately estimate parameters of interest or draw conclusions about the statistical significance of treatment effect based on a sparse sampling or reduced group size.

The methodology of choice for data analysis is the population approach, which is also known as non-linear mixed effects modelling. The

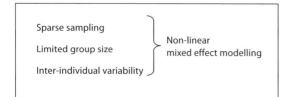

**Fig. 5.** Data analysis limitations due to small group size and sparse sampling can be overcome by the population approach. The method lends itself to the identification of the sources of inter-individual variability in pharmacokinetics and pharmacodynamics.

population approach allows characterisation of the sources of variability in drug concentrations or treatment response among individuals receiving clinically relevant doses of a drug of interest.

The use of the population approach to evaluate drug pharmacokinetics in the paediatric population is the subject of specific guidelines from the ICH, FDA and CHMP. Despite the focus of guidelines on pharmacokinetic studies, the population approach can be extended to the assessment of pharmacokinetic-pharmacodynamic relationships and efficacy (fig. 5).

Population pharmacokinetics seeks to identify the measurable pathophysiologic factors that cause changes in the dose-concentration relationship and the extent of these changes so that, if such changes are associated with clinically significant shifts in the therapeutic index, dosage can be appropriately modified. Patient demographics, pathophysiology and other therapeutic features, such as body weight, excretory and metabolic functions, and the presence of co-medication, can regularly alter dose-concentration relationships.

Using the population pharmacokinetic approach in drug development offers the possibility of gaining integrated information on pharmacokinetics, not only from relatively sparse data obtained from study subjects, but also from relatively dense data or a combination of sparse and dense data [8, 9]. The approach allows the analysis of data from a variety of unbalanced designs as well as from studies that are normally excluded because they do not lend themselves to the usual forms of pharmacokinetic analysis.

The use of the population approach for pharmacokinetic data analysis requires special consideration to be given to the following aspects in the study design:

- Where feasible, the study population, sample size, and age distribution should be adequate, either in a single study or several studies, to provide information on all the paediatric age groups for which the drug is intended.
- If other factors affecting the pharmacokinetics of the drug are to be studied (e.g. the effect of a concomitant medication or the presence or absence of a disease), sufficient numbers of subjects with and without the factor should be included in the study.
- The sampling scheme should be carefully planned to obtain the maximum information using the minimum number of samples.
- Some knowledge of the pharmacokinetics of the drug to be investigated from previous adult or paediatric experience may be used to develop the sampling scheme.

The following covariates should ordinarily be obtained for each subject: height, weight, body surface area, gestational age and birth weight for neonates, and relevant laboratory tests that reflect the function of organs responsible for drug elimination. Concomitant and recent drug therapy should also be recorded. The relationship between these parameters and the pharmacokinetics of the drug of interest should be examined using suitable statistical techniques and study designs.

In statistical terms, when evaluating relevant pharmacokinetic and pharmacodynamic parameters, one should assess whether the estimated parameters in children originates from a different distribution, as compared to the adult or other reference population.

*Additional Considerations*

*Adolescence*

In addition to puberty itself, several clinical specific elements should be considered. As an example, growth criteria may not be useful in pubertal populations. Furthermore, since endocrinological changes occur during puberty, they might influence clinical and biochemical parameters. In this age group non-adherence is high. Therefore, psychosocial interactions are already important in the planning phase.

*Pregnancy*

In most studies, pregnancy may interfere with study medication. In phase II/III studies usually pregnancy has to be excluded before study entry and has to be controlled during the study. The special problems of the study population have to be evaluated. Therefore, special reference with paediatric gynaecological expertise has to be encountered.

*Compliance/Adherence*

Non-compliance/adherence is of particular importance in all clinical studies. However, in the paediatric study population this depends not only on the patient but also on the parents (child caregiver). Patchwork families as well as families with a single caregiver are frequent. These specific situations need to be considered when planning paediatric clinical studies.

*Support from and Liaising with Paediatric Research Networks*

Many diseases in children have a low incidence, and only a multicentre approach makes recruitment of a sufficient number of patients possible. Paediatric research networks can support the realistic planning of clinical studies and help with their execution. Most subspecialties have a contact address with the Confederation of European Specialists in Paediatrics (CESP) that has recently took on the new name of European Academy of Paediatrics (EAP). CESP/EAP is part of the European Union of Medical Specialties (UEMS) of the member countries of the European Union (EU) and the European Free Trade Association (EFTA). It is governed by the provisions of these statutes, grouping together paediatricians without regard to their field, their mode of practice or their legal situation (www.cesp-eap.org). Several national paediatric research networks have been built up, such as PAED-Net in Germany (www.paed-net.org), the Dutch Medicines for Children Research Network (www.nkfk.nl), the UK Medicines for Children Research Network (www.mcrn.org.uk), and the Belgian Paediatric Research Network (www.pediatricdrug.be). These networks are prepared to help with strategic advice on paediatric development plans as well as with the support of executing individual studies. There is general agreement that study networks should be implemented in the European paediatric Societies. The future will tell to what degree these networks will be established.

## Conclusions

Responsibility for the study and protocol design for paediatric patients require not only solid knowledge of the methodology of adult clinical trials, but also in-depth understanding of child physiology, child psychology, the social embedding of children, the way institutions that take care of children work, and many other factors. It is rare that all this knowledge can be found within one single person. Usually, it requires a dedicated team with specialists in different specialties and a dedicated driver of the entire project. The execution of the study requires tight collaboration between academic researchers, industrial sponsors, and, if applicable, a dedicated clinical research organization.

## References

1   Stephenson T: How children's responses to drugs differ from adults. Br J Clin Pharmacol 2005;59:670–673.
2   Benedetti MS, Baltes EL: Drug metabolism and disposition in children. Fund Clin Pharmacol 2003;17:281–299.
3   Johnson TN, Rostami-Hodjegan A, Tucker GT: Prediction of the clearance of eleven drugs and associated variability in neonates, infants and children. Clin Pharmacokinet 2006;45:931–956.
4   Palmer CR: Ethics, data-dependent designs, and the strategy of clinical trials: time to start learning-as-we-go? Stat Methods Med Res 2002;11:381–402.
5   Holford N, Hashimoto Y, Sheiner LB: Time and theophylline concentration help explain the recovery of peak flow following acute airways obstruction: population analysis of a randomised concentration controlled trial. Clin Pharmacokinet 1993;25:506–515.
6   Giannini EH, Lovell DJ, Silverman ED, Sundel RP, Tague BL, Ruperto N: Intravenous immunoglobulin in the treatment of polyarticular juvenile rheumatoid arthritis: a phase I/II study. Pediatric Rheumatology Collaborative Study Group. J Rheumatol 1996;23:919–924.
7   Feldman B, Wang E, Willan A, Szalai JP: The randomized placebo-phase design for clinical trials. J Clin Epidemiol 2001;54:550–557.
8   Meibohm B, Läer S, Panetta JC 1st, Barrett JS: Population pharmacokinetic studies in pediatrics: issues in design and analysis. AAPS J 2005;7:E475–E487.
9   Knibbe CA, Zuideveld KP, DeJongh J, Kuks PF, Aarts LP, Danhof M: Population pharmacokinetic and pharmacodynamic modeling of propofol for long-term sedation in critically ill patients: a comparison between propofol 6% and propofol 1%. Clin Pharmacol Ther 2002;72:670–684.

Rose K, van den Anker JN (eds): Guide to Paediatric Clinical Research.
Basel, Karger, 2007, pp 108–114

··········

# Innovative Methodologies for Drug Evaluation in Children

*Gerard Pons*[a]   *John N. van den Anker*[b]

[a]University Rene Descartes, Clinical Pharmacology, Cochin –
Saint Vincent de Paul Hospital, Paris, France; [b]Division of Pediatric
Clinical Pharmacology, Children's National Medical Center, and
Departments of Pediatrics, Pharmacology and Physiology, George
Washington University School of Medicine and Health Sciences,
Washington, D.C., USA, and Department of Pediatrics, Erasmus MC –
Sophia Children's Hospital, Rotterdam, The Netherlands

## Introduction

Children are different because drugs behave differently in their bodies. The fate of drugs is different in the body of children as their pharmacokinetic parameters vary as a function of age with different maturational profiles regarding absorption, distribution, metabolism and elimination [1]. The effect of drugs is different in children as the magnitude of the response may differ and the nature of the response may also be different: some side effects only occur in children as their bodies undergo continuous growth and maturation. Children are also different because their diseases may be different as compared to adults. Some diseases only occur in children. Other diseases differ in nature from that observed in adults. Infectious diseases have different epidemiologies of the micro-organisms. Malignancies have different histological types, different prognosis, and different responses to drug therapy. Epilepsy has a higher incidence than in adults, various epileptic syndromes occurring in children are absent in adults, juvenile epilepsy has severe cognitive prognosis, a type of seizure may change with age, the syndromes may have different response to anti-epileptic drugs with possible worsening unlike in adults, some anti-epileptic side effects are specific to children [2, 3]. Not only are children different from adults but they represent a heterogeneous group in which due to the maturation different age classes had to be distinguished as they differ regarding drug fate and drug effect. Different main age classes have been defined by ICH E 11 [4].

This chapter describes the main issues to be faced when performing clinical studies in children and the methodological approaches that can be undertaken in an attempt to circumvent some of them.

## Invasiveness

Invasiveness of clinical studies is related to pain, stress, blood deprivation, and eventually exposure to radio-active isotopes. Exposure to clinical trials and to investigational new drugs should be limited to the minimum required.

To prevent pain and stress related to blood sampling in children the use of local anaesthesia (such as the use of EMLA cream) and of catheters to avoid repetitive venipunctures should be standard of care. The assessment of efficacy should be performed as much as possible through non-invasive procedures such as transcutaneous methods: $PO_2$, $PCO_2$, $SAO_2$, temperature, bilirubin, echodoppler (cerebral blood flow, heart, vessels), and neuroimaging, However, non-invasive methods have to be carefully validated to yield appropriate surrogate markers. To restrict blood loss, small blood samples should be drawn and micro-assays developed for appropriate assays with high sensitivity and specificity. To restrict blood loss a small number of blood samples per patient should be drawn. To perform pharmacokinetic (PK) and pharmacokinetic-pharmacodynamic (PK-PD) studies, the use of population approaches have to be developed. While a 'rich data' individual approach requires many blood samples in a few patients, population (POP) approaches (POP-PK) require fewer blood samples per patient in a larger number of patients. Alternative approaches such as saliva sampling may be misleading. Although a good correlation between saliva and plasma drug concentration has been shown for several drugs, the large scatter of the data points around the correlation line precludes in most cases appropriate estimation of a plasma concentration from the concomitant saliva concentration [5].

Irradiation by the use of radioactive compounds has to be avoided in children and the use of stable isotopes has to be stimulated. The use of the labelling of medicinal products by stable isotopes is of great potential interest in children for bioavailability studies, pharmacokinetic studies during repeated doses treatment, for metabolic studies, such as $CO_2$ breath test and for measuring compliance to the treatment [6].

Restricting exposure to clinical studies and to investigational new drugs whenever possible requires one to avoid unnecessary studies and the lowest possible age-limit to which adult data can be extrapolated should be determined; the already available paediatric data in the literature and data in the file should also be taken into account.

In order to extrapolate adult data to the lowest possible age limit in children, available data on the maturational profiles relevant to pharmacokinetics (renal elimination, metabolic pathways), to PK-PD (level of systemic exposure, minimum plasma concentration and area under the plasma concentration-time curve) and to safety (renal elimination, metabolism) are to be used. The knowledge of the ontogeny of the processes involved in drug elimination by indicating the lowest possible age limit for extrapolation from adults to children is very useful for planning paediatric pharmacokinetic studies allowing optimisation of age distribution in the recruitment of patients and for the numerical modelling of the influence of maturation allowing simulation of clinical trials [7].

Unnecessary studies can also be avoided by the use of other already available data: The bio-availability of paediatric formulations measured in healthy adult volunteers are to be used as a human model and only confirmation data are to be performed in children. Population pharmacokinetic analysis can sometimes be performed on published data avoiding the need to perform specific studies on the influence of maturation on pharmacokinetics in children [8]. Meta-analysis of already published data has to be performed whenever possible [9].

### Recruitment of Paediatric Patients

The recruitment of children is more difficult than in adults: the number of available patients is often limited and informed consent is more difficult to obtain than in adults and exposure to clinical studies and investigational new drugs has to be limited to the minimum. A balance is to be found between the ethical issue on the one hand pushing at using the smallest possible numbers of patients to recruit and on the other hand the validity of scientific data as well as the acceptance by regulatory bodies of the studies for the application of marketing authorization pushing for the numbers of patients not to be too small. Innovative methodological approaches can be used to restrict the number of patients to be included in clinical studies.

Sequential approaches can be used for dose-finding studies in phase II as well as for comparative trials in phase III:

- Dose-finding parallel group studies are difficult to perform in children due to the relatively narrow dose range and the small interval between tested doses, the important inter-individual variability of the parameters measured and therefore the lack of statistical power that could theoretically be increased by enlarging the number of patients recruited. A new promising method, the continual re-assessment method (CRM), has been proposed and used in several instances in children [10–13]. This method has the advantage of not requiring a placebo group, and that each new patient is receiving a dose closer to the optimal dose. This method requires only a limited number of patients (15–20). The flaws of the method are that it requires qualitative parameters, rapid evaluation of the response and a very efficient organisation.
- Sequential approaches such as the triangular test are of great potential interest in phase III comparative clinical trials in that they allow one to recruit a smaller number of patients as the study can be stopped as soon as sufficient information to conclude the study has been collected [14].

Responder population enrichment has been used to decrease the variability of the response increasing the statistical power in order to facilitate the demonstration of efficacy.

Clinical trial numerical modelling and in silico simulation is a promising avenue to explore.

Strategies using appropriate methodological approaches are to be developed for the measurement of drug effect for unpredicted late toxicity on developing organs and to be used in post-marketing studies are of particular interest in children. Therapeutic catastrophies of the past such as the retrolental fibroplasia related to oxygen exposure, phocomelia related to thalidomide, adenocarcinoma of the vagina after intra-uterine exposure to diethylstilboestrol and more recent findings such as delayed cardiac toxicity of anthracyclins, delayed testicular toxicity of Hodgkin-'MOPP' chemotherapy, delayed ovarian toxicity of high doses of busulfan before BMT, and premature ovarian failure in cancer survivors showed that exposure to medicinal products during growth and maturation from conception to adulthood may severely impact on these biological processes and may only become apparent with delay [15–19]. Long-term prospective follow-up studies on growth and maturation, reproductive capacity, ability to learn, and emotional and psychological development are to be performed in children seeking for side effects that occur far beyond the period of drug exposure. Appropriate methodological approaches have to be used in this matter: case studies nested in cohort studies are of particular potential interest in children.

## Specific Tools

Appropriate tools have to be developed for the measurement of drug effect because children do not express their distress in the same way as adults. Appropriate scales for measuring the magnitude of response to medicinal products had to be developed for pain and have for example to be further developed for sedation and muscular strength. Similarly, new clinical and biological end-points and surrogate markers have to be validated in children. For instance, the visual analogue scale, a validated tool in adults, cannot reliably be used under the age of 6 years. Face scales, 'poker chips' are used between 4 and 6 years. Below the age of 6 years most often pain and the effect of analgesic agents cannot be measured using auto-evaluation but only by hetero-evaluation. The scales for pain and the evaluation of analgesic drugs under the age of 6 years not only vary according to age but also according to the clinical condition such as post-operative pain: Objective Pain Scale (OPS) above 2 months of age, Children's Hospital of Eastern Ontario Pain scale

1 year of age, Amiel-Tison scale between 1 month and 3 years of age. In other acute pain situations, the CHEOPS scale may also be used but in the neonate specific scales have to be developed such as the Neonatal Facial Coding System (NFCS). For long-lasting pain the behaviour of children is completely different and acute pain scales can no longer be used and specific scales have to be developed such as the DEGR scale (between 2 and 6 years of age) and the EDIN scale for premature neonates. So, the appropriate tools for the measurement of the efficacy of analgesic agent not only vary with age but also with clinical conditions [20].

Innovative methodologies are potential useful tools to facilitate drug evaluation in children whenever necessary. They are not expected to replace classical approaches. The limits of validity of these approaches are to be evaluated for appropriate level of evidence of efficacy and safety. Due to the constraints of drug evaluation in children paediatric clinical pharmacology represents a challenging area for methodological creativity which may ultimately give benefit to other areas of clinical pharmacology including to adults.

## References

1   Kearns GL, Abdel-Rahman SM, Alander SW, Blowey DL, Leeder JS, Kauffman RE: Developmental pharmacology: drug disposition, action, and therapy in infants and children. N Engl J Med 2003;349:1157–1167.
2   Commission on Classification and Terminology of the International League Against Epilepsy: Proposal for revised classification of epilepsies and epileptic syndromes. Epilepsia 1989;30:389–399.
3   Guerrini R, Dravet C, Genton P, Belmonte A, Kaminska A, Dulac O: Lamotrigine and seizure aggravation in severe myoclonic epilepsy. Epilepsia 1998;39:508–512.
4   ICH Topic E 11: Clinical Investigation of medicinal products in the paediatric population. Note for guidance on clinical investigation of medicinal products in the paediatric population (CPMP/ICH/2711/99). http://www.emea.eu.int/pdfs/human/ich/271199en.pdf
5   Gao Y, Pons G, Rey E, Richard MO, d'Athis P, Bertin L, Thiroux G, de Blic J, Scheinmann P, Olive G: Could saliva stand for plasma in theophylline monitoring in asthmatic children? Still a controversial problem. Fundam Clin Pharmacol 1992;6:191–196.
6   Pons G, Rey E: Stable isotopes labeling of drugs in pediatric clinical pharmacology. Pediatrics 1999;104:633–639.
7   Johnson TN: Modelling approaches to dose estimation in children. Br J Clin Pharmacol 2005;59:663–669.
8   Anderson BJ, Pons G, Autret-Leca E, Allegaert K, Boccard E: Pediatric intravenous paracetamol (propacetamol) pharmacokinetics: a population analysis. Paediatr Anaesth 2005;15:282–292.

9   Kassaî B, Chiron C, Guerrini R, Augier S, Cucherat M, Rey E, Gueyffier F, Dulac O, Vincent J, Pons G: Stiripentol and severe myoclonic epilepsy in infancy: a systematic review and a meta-analysis of individual patient data. Epilepsia (under revision).

10  Desfrere L, Zohar S, Morville P, Brunhes A, Chevret S, Pons G, Moriette G, Rey E, Treluyer JM: Dose-finding study of ibuprofen in patent ductus arteriosus using the continual reassessment method. J Clin Pharm Ther 2005;30:121–132.

11  de Spirlet M, Treluyer JM, Chevret S, Rey E, Tournaire M, Cabrol D, Pons G: Toco-lytic effects of intravenous nitroglycerin. Fundam Clin Pharmacol 2004;18:207–213.

12  Treluyer JM, Zohar S, Rey E, Hubert P, Iserin F, Jugie M, Lenclen R, Chevret S, Pons G: Minimum effective dose of midazolam for sedation of mechanically ventilated ne-onates. J Clin Pharm Ther 2005;30:479–485.

13  Fabre E, Chevret S, Piechaud JF, Rey E, Vauzelle-Kervoedan F, D'Athis P, Olive G, Pons G: An approach for dose finding of drugs in infants: sedation by midazolam studied using the continual reassessment method. Br J Clin Pharmacol 1998;46:395–401.

14  Bellissant E, Duhamel JF, Guillot M, Pariente-Khayat A, Olive G, Pons G: The trian-gular test to assess the efficacy of metoclopramide in gastroesophageal reflux. Clin Pharmacol Ther 1997;61:377–384.

15  Teinturier C, Hartmann O, Valteau-Couanet D, Benhamou E, Bougneres PF: Ovarian function after autologous bone marrow transplantation in childhood: high-dose bu-sulfan is a major cause of ovarian failure. Bone Marrow Transplant 1998;22:989–994.

16  Lipshultz SE: Exposure to anthracyclines during childhood causes cardiac injury. Semin Oncol 2006;33(3 suppl 8):S8–S14.

17  Brice P: Cured from Hodgkin's disease. Bull Cancer 2002;89:666–670.

18  Chen WY, Manson JE: Premature Ovarian Failure in Cancer Survivors: New Insights, Looming concerns. J Natl Cancer Inst, 2006;98:880–881.

19  Stinson JN, Kavanagh T, Yamada J, Gill N, Stevens B: Systematic review of the psycho-metric properties, interpretability and feasibility of self. Pain 2006.

20  Hobbie WL, Ginsberg JP, Ogle SK, Carlson CA, Meadows AT: Fertility in males treat-ed for Hodgkins disease with COPP/ABV hybrid. Pediatr Blood Cancer 2005;44:193–196.

Rose K, van den Anker JN (eds): Guide to Paediatric Clinical Research.
Basel, Karger, 2007, pp 115–125

......................

# Challenges in the Research of Very Small Children

*John N. van den Anker*[a]   *José Ramet*[b]

[a]Division of Pediatric Clinical Pharmacology, Children's National Medical
Center, and Departments of Pediatrics, Pharmacology and Physiology,
George Washington University School of Medicine and Health Sciences,
Washington, D.C., USA, and Department of Pediatrics, Erasmus MC –
Sophia Children's Hospital, Rotterdam, The Netherlands; [b]University
of Antwerp, Universitair Ziekenhuis Antwerpen UZA and ZNA,
Paola Children's Hospital, Antwerp, Belgium

The history of drug therapy shows that newborn infants are more prone to experience adverse reactions to medicines. In 1956, Silverman et al. [1] reported an excessive mortality rate and an increased incidence of kernicterus among preterm neonates receiving a sulfonamide antibiotic as compared to neonates receiving chlortetracycline. Then, in 1959, Sutherland [2] described a syndrome of cardiovascular collapse in newborns receiving high doses of chloramphenicol for presumed infections. More recently, the therapeutic misadventures experienced by low-birthweight infants exposed to a parenteral vitamin E formulation [3] and the 'gasping syndrome' by infants who received excessive amount of benzyl alcohol [4, 5] underscore the persistence of problems with the use of medicines in neonates. As a result of these experiences neonatologists and paediatricians have recognized that rational drug therapy for neonates is often confounded by a combination of unpredictable and often poorly understood pharmacokinetic and pharmacodynamic interactions [6–9]. A more specific approach to neonatal therapeutics requires a thorough understanding of human developmental biology as well as insights regarding the dynamic ontogeny of the processes of drug absorption, drug distribution, drug metabolism, and drug excretion. Many excellent reviews on this topic are currently available and will therefore not be the focus of this chapter [10, 11]. It is clear that more clinical trials are needed to study the effects of medicines in very small infants and to improve evidence-based pharmacotherapy in this group of vulnerable patients. It is not easy, however, to conduct pharmacological studies in these patients. Therefore, this chapter will focus on neonates as an example of a very small infant population and will explore some of the issues that may complicate neonatal clinical trials and gives recommendations for randomised controlled trials (RCTs) in neonates in general.

## Introduction

With a substantial body of knowledge and evidence still missing, only few neonatal pharmacological trials are available. Therefore, neonates often are given medicines without any license or in an 'off-label' fashion [12]. Since the FDA Modernization Act (FDAMA) was signed into law in 1997 the US National Institute of Health and the Food and Drug Administration have undertaken initiatives to delineate this problem and to develop a research agenda to study drugs in newborn infants. However, many hurdles have to be taken before a well-designed neonatal trial can be conducted. First of all, hospital ethics committees may be reluctant to agree with drug trials in very small infants. Secondly, it may be challenging to obtain parental informed consent. Finally, it may be very difficult to get funding for trials investigating the use of off-patent drugs.

Yet there are pressing arguments to study the effects of medicines in neonates. We cannot just base dosing regimens on schedules derived from adults and even from children, as the pharmacokinetics and dynamics of drugs in premature neonates are quite different [13]. Therefore, drug trials in neonates are essential to determine optimal drug dosing regimens in this age group [14].

Trials in neonates vary from early phase II to phase III trials. Ideally, the latter will have full-scale evaluation, comparing current standard treatment (using a control group) with the new drug. To prevent biased evaluation of the new treatment, each patient is randomly assigned to either new or standard treatment. Trials are then randomized controlled trials (RCTs), which are considered best for research [15].

However, before being able to conduct these important phase III trials there need to be information about the appropriate dose to be used for these investigations. Thus, there is an apparent need for studies that will define the right doses for different gestational and postnatal ages. These dosing regimens need to take into account general developmental changes in metabolism and renal clearance on the one hand and the individual patient's pharmacogenetic background on the other hand.

## Teamwork

Meeting the quality requirements – from designing the study protocol up to publication of the results – needs multidisciplinary team involvement. Crucially, successful completion of the study requires all players be involved from the start. It will not work at all, for example, to exclude the statistician until all data have been collected. In addition to the principal investigator, such a team would typically consist of nurses, neonatologists, a developmental pharmacologist, a psychologist, a methodologist, a biostatistician, a pharmacist and a clinical chemist. The role of the pharmacist is important. The test drugs and placebo must have a similar appearance. Furthermore, the pharmacy might perform the randomization.

## CONSORT Statements and Registration of Trials

Evidently, all team members should be familiar with the CONSORT guidelines [16] and ultimately the study protocol should comply with these guidelines. Using the CONSORT guidelines as a checklist helps to consider issues which otherwise could be overlooked, such as follow-up of refusals, adequate description of randomization and blinding. Furthermore, peer-reviewed journals with high impact factors require trials to conform to the CONSORT guidelines. This may stimulate uniformity in reporting RCTs.

The International Committee of Medical Journal Editors (ICMJE) recently ruled that for trials to be published, subscription into a public trials registry (http://www.clinicaltrials.gov/) at or before start of patient enrolment is required as from July 2005 [17]. This measure is expected to reduce publication bias, the tendency that non-significant or 'less interesting' results are less likely to be published than are significant results. Paediatric trials may be entered into the Drug Evaluation in Children register (www.dec-net.org). The DEC-net Register is supported under the European Union's Fifth Framework programme 'Quality of Life', and was activated on July 1, 2004.

## Pilot Study

Once a study protocol has been created, its practical execution may present unforeseen problems. For instance, it may be far too optimistic with regards to number of patients included and speed of inclusion. This may be problematic and challenging as studies are often sponsored by grants of limited duration. A pilot study may give an estimation of required sample size and facilitates a realistic power analysis. In addition, a pilot study may reveal logistic or practical problems and provides for instrument testing and improvement of task allocation, etc. It does not solve all obstacles, as was seen in one of our studies in preterm infants [18]. While the pilot study had raised high expectations about patient inclusion, we were confronted with a refusal rate as high as 28% in the RCT (fig. 1). In this study we concluded that it was due to obtain informed consent within 8 h after the start of mechanical ventilation, when parents are often still in shock from the preterm delivery of their infants.

## Communication

It may seem obvious, but continuous communication between team members, parents and NICU staff throughout the study is crucial. Parents will highly appreciate receiving a report stating the most relevant results of the study afterwards. It should also be always clear who has final responsibility for trial participants.

Close collaboration between medical and nursing staff is highly important. Nurses and medical staff may present difficulties if they are not

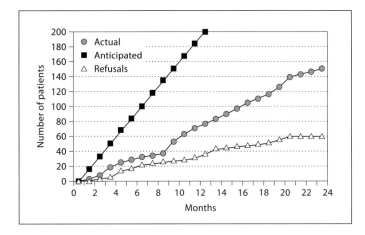

*Fig. 1.* Comparison of actual and planned inclusion of patients in the NICU pain study.

convinced of the value of the research project. In this case, they may have less appreciation of the study's relevance. Special meetings that address these questions and newsletters can help improve communication and collaboration.

Some members of ethical committees, staff members and others are still of the opinion that small patients need protection against research. The better these concerns are addressed, the more they will be prepared to collaborate.

Finally, in multi-centre studies research meetings with all collaborating centres are crucial to guarantee study protocol adherence.

## Consent

Communication with parents is challenging at the start of the study when informed consent is sought, and the more so if the study protocol dictates well-timed enrolment soon after birth. Parents who are still in shock because their child was born preterm and is in a severe disease state such as meconium aspiration syndrome or congenital anomalies may be inclined to refuse consent. This hurdle may be overcome in part by having the attending neonatologist explain the study antenatally, when parents are not exhausted and upset [19, 20]. However, this remedy is of little help in the often unexpected preterm or complicated deliveries. A more preferable option is to have the clinical researchers and not the treating neonatologist ask consent independently to avoid (suspicion of) conflict of interest. Valid informed consent suggests that parents understand the purpose of the study as well as its benefits and risks. In addition they should be aware of the voluntary nature of their participation. Mason et al. [21] reported the lack of *valid* informed consent from 71.5% of 200 parents who had been asked consent for inclusion of their neonates in a trial. Problems were related to non-understanding, involuntariness, incompetence and information problems. Ballard et al. [22] recently found that only 5% of 64 parents understood any potential risk from participating in the NEOPAIN study in which neonates received 10–30 µg morphine/kg/h or placebo. These examples show that devising the best possible strategy of asking parental consent is quite essential. Table 1 summarizes some of the issues and solutions in the consent process.

## Use of Placebo

It can be debated if neonates can experience a placebo effect of drug therapy. Giving no placebo can, however, bias those who measure the effect of pharmacological interventions. As placebo is required to ensure blinding during the trial, inclusion of a placebo group into the study design is warranted even in neonatal trials. It may be appropriate to use a placebo if the efficacy of an analgesic drug has not been proven in a specific clinical situation. However, placebo is only an option for the control group when there is no existing standard drug therapy against which the new drug should be compared. The World Medical Association has developed the Declaration of Helsinki as a statement of ethical principles to provide guidance to physicians and other participants in medical research involving human subjects.

The use of placebo in trials was first mentioned in the 1996 version. The latest version (2000) includes a clause 29 stating: *'The benefits, risks, burdens and effectiveness of a new method should be tested against those of the best current prophylactic, diagnostic, and therapeutic methods. This does not exclude the use of placebo, or no treatment, in studies where no*

**Table 1.** Some issues and possible solutions around informed consent

| Issues | Possible solutions |
|--------|--------------------|
| Time pressure, emergency research*, less than 24 h reflection time for parents | give antenatal information and ask presumed consent (with possibility of opting out) or adapt research question and protocol including more time before inclusion |
| Parents are in shock and cannot properly decide | antenatal information with presumed consent and possibility of opting out |
| No full understanding of procedure, benefits and risks associated with study, right to withdraw from study at any time | both oral and written information and check if information was understood; point out that an independent neonatologist is available for consultation |
| Parents feel pressure/ involuntariness | researcher, and not attending physician, should ask consent |

* Intervention must take place within 24 h.

*proven prophylactic, diagnostic or therapeutic method exists.'* This seemed to rule out the use of placebo wherever proven treatment existed. In reaction to protests from the medical world, in 2001 a Note of Clarification was added to Clause 29, describing the circumstances when a placebo-controlled trial is acceptable even if proven therapy is available [23].

### Dose Regimen

One of the most important issues in designing a drug trial is probably the determination of the dose regimen of the investigated drug. Effective doses (per kg body weight) vary with changing gestational and postnatal ages. Optimal dosing regimens should be based on extensive literature reviews. In general it is a matter of balancing between high doses that are effective and low doses that cause no adverse effects. Another consideration, aimed at avoiding staff uneasiness, is using doses that approximate those that were standard of care before the trial started.

To find the appropriate dose to be used in randomized controlled trials, a pharmacokinetic study needs to be designed that will use the least amount of blood samples to arrive at the correct dose recommendation. For scientific investigations in neonates ethical review boards will typically allow the use of maximal 3 ml/kg of blood. In other words, for a preterm infant of 800 g a total of 2.4 ml may be used for both the pharmacokinetic analysis and the safety labs surrounding the exposure to the investigational drug. Evidently, we need precise microanalytical assays that will allow us to do these studies. The use of HPLC assays and more recently HPLC-MS/MS techniques have revolutionized the opportunities for even the smallest prematurely born neonates. A recent development is the application of sparse pharmacokinetic sampling in larger neonatal populations to better describe pharmacokinetics using population analysis approaches. In this analysis approach, some precision in the pharmacokinetic parameters of individual participants is sacrificed by taking fewer samples to allow inclusion of a wider spectrum of participants likely to receive the drug clinically. Although reduction in frequency and number of samples has obvious appeal in neonatal populations, the ability of population methods to analyze unbalanced data collected at various time points is also attractive in these populations. This method allows pooling of data across studies to provide a uniform, robust, single pharmacokinetic analysis rather than attempting to compare results of separate, smaller studies that are complicated by significant analysis methodology differences.

## Toxicity

Apart from positive effects, such as analgesia or stress relief, drugs may cause toxicity. Toxicity denotes either the capacity of the studied drug to cause harm to a living organism, or the occurrence of adverse effects caused by a chemical. Hard to predict, toxicity may result from overdosing or from idiosyncratic reactions of individual patients such as hepatic or kidney failure or pharmacokinetic/pharmacogenetic profile. As only few patients may show adverse effects, trials which focus on side effects should have large sample size for sufficient power. Adverse effects known to result from certain drugs should be monitored at predetermined time-points. This may be a challenge.

### Rescue Medication

Administration of rescue medication in RCTs is primarily guided by the subjective clinical judgment of staff present at the time.

The use of an algorithm including decision rules for the administration of rescue medication would enhance objectivity and standardisation of treatment. However, the very administration of rescue medication may complicate the statistical analysis and diminish the strength of the study design, especially when rescue medication is required frequently.

As rescue medication reflects normal clinical practice, a study design that provides for the use of rescue medication is preferred. However, in analysing the results one should be aware of the problem of 'the dog biting its own tail', i.e. high pain scores (outcome) may be linked with the use of rescue medication (outcome as well). This problem complicates studies aiming to determine the analgesic effect of a drug. In such studies the amount of rescue medication might be used as a covariate.

### Multiple Centres Involved: Many Differences

In order to obtain sufficient sample size and to increase the power of the results, multi-centre trials seem to be the answer. Multi-centre trials, however, have drawbacks. All logistical problems of single-centre RCTs are even more apparent in large multi-centre trials. Furthermore, formalities, such as who is funding the research, whose name is on the published manuscripts, may be required. Then there are statistical considerations in that observations within centres may be correlated [24]. Failure to consider the centre in statistical analysis may result firstly in incorrect p values and confidence intervals. Secondly, biased estimates may present themselves because of uncontrolled confounding. For instance, if proportions of very premature neonates vary between centres and this variation affects treatment as well as the outcome, confounding is apparent. Thirdly, effect modification may occur if the effect of treatment on outcome varies significantly between centres. This effect could be efficiently tested for example by random-coefficient models [24].

## Conclusion

Studies in neonates of different gestational and postnatal ages are needed to assure safe and effective pharmacotherapy for this most vulnerable patient population. Several challenges discussed in this chapter are surmountable and will guarantee optimal designed studies that will improve the mortality and morbidity of these very small children.

## References

1 Silverman WA, Anderson DH, Blanc WA, et al: A difference in mortality rate and incidence of kernicterus among premature infants allotted to two prophylactic antibacterial regimens. Pediatrics 1956;18:614–624.
2 Sutherland JM: Fatal cardiovascular collapse of infants receiving large amount of chloramphenicol. Am J Dis Child 1959;97:761–767.
3 Lorch V, Murphy D, Hoersten LR, Harris E, Fitzgerald J, Sinha SN: Unusual syndrome among premature infants: association with a new intravenous vitamin E product. Pediatrics 1985;75:598–602.
4 Lovejoy FH: Benzyl alcohol poisoning in neonatal intensive care units. A new concern for the pediatrician. Am J Dis Child 1982;136:974–975.
5 Christensen ML, Helms RA, Chesney RW: Is pediatric labeling really necessary? Pediatrics 1999;104(suppl):593–597.
6 Lobstein R, Koren G: Clinical relevance of therapeutic drug monitoring during pregnancy. Ther Drug Monit 2002;24:15–22.
7 Garland M: Pharmacology of drug transfer across the placenta. Obstet Gynecol Clin N Am 1998;25:21–42.
8 Berlin CM Jr: Advances in pediatric pharmacology and toxicology. Adv Pediatr 1997; 44:545–574.
9 Kearns GL: Impact of developmental pharmacology on pediatric study design: overcoming the challenges. J Allergy Clin Immunol 2000;106(3 suppl):S128–S138.
10 Kearns GL, Abdel-Rahman SM, Alander SW, Blowey DL, Leeder JS, Kauffman RE: Developmental Pharmacology – drug disposition, action and therapy in infants and children. N Engl J Med 2003;349:1157-1167.
11 Rakhmanina NY, van den Anker JN: Pharmacological research in pediatrics: from neonates to adolescents. Adv Drug Deliv Rev 2006;58:4-14.
12 Choonara I: Unlicensed and off-label drug use in children: implications for safety. Expert Opin Drug Saf 2004;3:81–83.
13 Lingen van RA, Simons SHP, Anderson BJ, Tibboel D: The effects of analgesia in the vulnerable infant during the perinatal period. Clin Perinatol 2002;29:511–534.
14 Choonara I: Why do babies cry? We still know too little about what will ease babies' pain. BMJ 1999;319:1381.
15 Pocock SJ: Clinical Trials: A Practical Approach. Chichester, Wiley, 1983.
16 Moher D, Jones A, Lepage L: Use of the CONSORT statement and quality of reports of randomized trials: a comparative before-and-after evaluation. JAMA 2001;285:1992–1995.

17  DeAngelis CD, Drazen JM, Frizelle FA, et al: Clinical trial registration: a statement from the International Committee of Medical Journal Editors. JAMA 2004;292:1363–1364.

18  Simons SH, van Dijk M, van Lingen RA, et al: Routine morphine infusion in preterm newborns who received ventilatory support: a randomized controlled trial. JAMA 2003;290:2419–2427.

19  Burgess E, Singhal N, Amin H, McMillan DD, Devrome H: Consent for clinical research in the neonatal intensive care unit: a retrospective survey and a prospective study. Arch Dis Child Fetal Neonatal Ed 2003;88:F280–F285; discussion F285–F286.

20  Manning DJ: Presumed consent in emergency neonatal research. J Med Ethics 2000; 26:249–253.

21  Mason SA, Allmark PJ: Obtaining informed consent to neonatal randomised controlled trials: interviews with parents and clinicians in the Euricon study. Lancet 2000; 356:2045–2051.

22  Ballard HO, Shook LA, Desai NS, Anand KJ: Neonatal research and the validity of informed consent obtained in the perinatal period. J Perinatol 2004;24:409–415.

23  Carlson RV, Boyd KM, Webb DJ: The revision of the Declaration of Helsinki: past, present and future. Br J Clin Pharmacol 2004;57:695–713.

24  Localio AR, Berlin JA, Ten Have TR, Kimmel SE: Adjustments for center in multicenter studies: an overview. Ann Intern Med 2001;135:112–123.

Rose K, van den Anker JN (eds): Guide to Paediatric Clinical Research.
Basel, Karger, 2007, pp 126–132

··························

# Clinical Research for Infant Nutrition

*P. Steenhout*[a]   *E.E. Ziegler*[b]

[a]Nestlé Nutrition, Nestec Ltd., Vevey, Switzerland;
[b]Department of Pediatrics, University of Iowa, Iowa City, Iowa, USA

## Historical Background of Industrially Produced Baby Food

During the first months of life breastfeeding is the preferred feeding mode for infants. WHO recommends [1] that babies should be breastfed exclusively during the 6 first months of life. High-quality complementary feedings should be added beginning at 6 months of age. There are very few situations where, because of maternal or infant health concerns, breastfeeding is not recommended. When breastfeeding is not possible, or is not chosen by the parents, the use of breast milk substitutes (formulas) is required.

Infant formulas based on cow's milk were developed during the last decades of the 19th century and the early decades of the 20th century. During the remainder of the 20th century, efforts were mainly concentrated on improving infant formulas so they would more and more resemble breast milk, and produce responses in the infant similar to those of the breastfed infant. The result of these efforts are contemporary formulas that use cow milk essentially only as the source of protein and lactose, with all other components being derived from other sources.

Towards the end of the 20th century a new wave of innovations began which continues today. The use of new ingredients, including but not limited to Lc-Pufas, nucleotides, new combinations of cow milk protein fractions, prebiotics, probiotics and hydrolyzed proteins was explored and ultimately adopted. Also, the addition of proteins produced by recombinant techniques (e.g. lactoferrin) was begun and has offered unprecedented possibilities.

All innovations require extensive clinical testing in infants. It would be highly irresponsible to bring novel products with new components to market without support from extensive studies establishing the safety and efficacy of the novel products. Clinical testing is an essential part of formula development. Advances such as have been made in recent years would not be possible without clinical testing at every step.

## Regulatory Basis Pertaining to Infant Nutrition Products

The purpose of regulations is dual: (1) protect the consumer, and (2) organize free trade. Safety and efficacy are key aspects of regulations assessing infant nutrition products. Regulations lay down compositional criteria, provisions concerning food additives and labeling instructions.

On a global level, the Codex Alimentarius [2] sets the regulatory basis for infant nutrition. Codex Alimentarius has adopted an infant formula standard (Codex Stan 72-1981), which is currently under revision. The Codex infant formula standard has been adopted by many countries into their national regulations, or, in the absence of local regulations, is referred to by default.

In the US, infant nutrition regulations are codified in the Infant Formula Act, which is part of the Code of Federal Regulations (CFR 107) and enforced by the Food and Drug Administration (FDA) [3]. Prior to placement on the market of an infant formula, the FDA must be notified, who reserves for 90 days the right to raise objections.

In the European Union (EU), all member states comply with the infant formula and follow-on formula directive (91/321/EC), which is currently under revision. Member states can request justification from the formula manufacturer concerning the scientific evidence of a specific infant formula. At the EU level the scientific evaluation is conducted by the European Food Security Authority (EFSA – http://www.efsa.europa. eu/). Additionally, independent food safety authorities are established in EU member states, e.g. Afssa, Agence française de la sécurité sanitaire des aliments, in France (http://www.afssa.fr/), or the FSA, Food Standards Agency, in the UK (http://www.food.gov.uk/). The scientific opinions issued by EFSA and/or national food safety authorities form the basis for decisions by the European Commission and/or national authorities.

Although regulations concerning infant nutrition products generally pertain to healthy infants, as more and more products have been developed by industry for infants with specific diseases, regulations pertaining specifically to such products have been developed. For example, FSMP (food for specific medical purpose) and recommendations for premature babies were also recently issued [4].

## Development and Marketing of New Products

The development of new products is always driven by advances in food technology and by changes in scientific concepts. In the case of foods for infants, an additional driving force is the desire to mimic mother's milk as closely as possible. Regulatory authorities require extensive data before authorizing the marketing of new products for infants, including data from clinical trials. Rules and recommendations for the assessment infant formulas have been issued by authoritative bodies. One of the most complete set of guidelines has been issued by the UK Department of Health [5].

More recently ESPGHAN's Committee on Nutrition has issued position papers entitled 'The Nutritional and Safety Assessment of Breast Milk Substitutes and Other Dietary Products for Infants' [6] and 'Core Data for Nutrition Trials in Infants' [7].

## Specific Aspects of Clinical Trials Supporting New Infant Nutrition Products

All clinical trials regardless of the subjects to whom they pertain must follow the Good Clinical Practice rules as defined by the International Conference on Harmonisation of Technical Requirements for Registration of Pharmaceuticals for Human Use [8] and the Good Laboratory Practice rules [9] and must strictly adhere to the ethical rules defined by the Declaration of Helsinki [10]. There are no inherent reasons why infant nutrition trials should be exempt from any of these well established rules.

Infant nutrition trials differ in several aspects from trials involving pharmaceutical products.

- Under no circumstances must infant nutrition trials interfere with breast feeding or discourage mothers from breastfeeding.
- With the exception of products for specific medical purposes, infant nutrition trials must be conducted with normal healthy infants.
- During the first few months of life, infant nutrition products (formulas) are generally the sole or predominant source of nutrition. Criteria for nutritional and safety characterization infant formulas intended for the first few months of life are therefore more strict than criteria applied to products, mostly those intended for older infants that provide only a fraction of the total diet.
- It is now well recognized that early nutrition may have long-term consequences. Therefore, the evaluation of breast milk substitutes needs to consider also long-term nutritional and safety outcomes.
- Even for studies using a randomized double-blind design, inclusion of a breast-fed reference group is highly recommended for safety evaluation of infant formulas. Alternatively, the growth performance of trial infants may be assessed on the basis of the new WHO growth charts [11] that are based exclusively on breastfed infants.

### Examples of Infant Nutrition Studies

*Safety Studies*
As already mentioned, to establish the nutritional adequacy and safety of a new infant formula, safety studies are required. If the composition of the new formula differs substantially from products already on the market, more than one study will be needed. Preferably, those studies should be conducted in different locations (centres or countries).

In a typical study, normal term infants whose parents have decided not to breastfeed, are enrolled during the first 2 weeks of life. The study is conducted in randomized double-blind fashion and growth of the subjects is monitored until 4 months of age or longer. Generally, a product already on the market serves as control product.

The primary outcome is weight gain per day from enrolment to 4 months of age.

To demonstrate equivalence, it is generally agreed that mean weight gain should not differ by more than 3 g/day. The population variance (SD) for weight gain from two weeks to 4 months of age is about 4.5 g/day [12]. Therefore, to detect a difference in weight gain of 3.0 g/day between study groups at alpha = 0.05 and beta = 0.2 requires a minimum of 28 subjects of each sex in each treatment group.

*Efficacy Studies*

Efficacy studies are conducted in order to assess the efficacy of novel formula components in bringing about expected health effects. Examples of formula components that have been extensively tested in recent years include long-chain polyunsaturated fatty acids (Lc-Pufa), probiotics and prebiotics. Medical or nutritional claims may only be made if they are supported by data from efficacy studies. Generally, efficacy studies are conducted on healthy subjects. Because the effects tend to be modest in size, the number of subjects needed is high. Unfortunately, the number of subjects needed is often underestimated and studies therefore have insufficient statistical power. This explains why studies sometimes come to opposite conclusions regarding the efficacy of ingredients. More and more meta-analysis is used to overcome the problem of insufficient statistical power of individual studies.

An instructive example of this problem is the inconsistency in the demonstration of efficacy of the addition of Lc-Pufa to formulas for normal infants. Although it is well established that the addition of Lc-Pufa to formulas for premature infants is effective in improving visual acuity and brain development of premature babies, such effects have not been shown unequivocally in term infants.

In infants older than 6 months the difficulties in establishing efficacy are greater than in younger infants because the increasing consumption of complementary foods diversifies the infant's diet and introduces many confounding factors.

Finally, assessment of possible long-term effects of early feeding will require prospective longitudinal studies of unprecedented size (subject numbers) and complexity. It is possible that early biological markers (such as serum IGF-1 or C-peptide) may some day serve as surrogates for long-term outcomes. But then the establishment of early markers as valid predictors of late outcomes would require very larger and complex studies.

### Comparative Studies

Comparative studies are designed to demonstrate the equivalence or the superiority of a new concept or a new product. The comparison product may be a competitor's product. Such studies are mainly conducted with therapeutic nutritional products, including premature formulas.

### Tolerance Studies

Tolerance studies are necessary to test new ingredients for their suitability for use in infant nutrition products. Tolerance studies are also necessary to determine the level of a new ingredient that produces the desired efficacy while at the same time producing no or acceptable negative effects. Statistically, an adaptive two-stage design with sample size reassessment is particularly suitable for such studies. It permits early identification of adverse effects and continuation of the study with only those ingredient levels that are free of adverse effects.

## Conclusions

Clinical studies in infants are essential for the development and advancement of infant nutrition products. Studies must be carefully designed and have adequate statistical power in order to yield unequivocal answers. Studies must observe the same rules as pharmaceutical studies and use similar methodology. In addition, the design of infant nutrition studies must take into account certain unique considerations, such as the breastfed infant as a reference, food diversification, and possible long-term effects of early feeding.

## References

1  WHO 54th World Health Assembly: Infant and Young Child Nutrition. WHA 2001; 54.2.
2  Joint FAO/WHO Food Standards Programme Codex Alimentarius Commission: Food for special dietary uses (including foods for infants and children). Codex Alimentarius 1994;4.
3  Current Legislation and Regulations for Infant Formulas; in Kleinman RE (ed): Pediatric Nutrition Handbook. New York, American Academy of Pediatrics, 2004, pp 545–548.
4  Klein CJ: Nutrient requirements for preterm infant formulas. J Nutr 2002;132:1395S–1577S.
5  Guidelines on the Nutritional Assessment of Infant Formulas: Report on Health and Social Subjects. London, UK Department of Health – The Stationery Office, 1996, p 47.
6  Aggett P, Agostini C, Goulet O, Hernell O, Koletzko B, Lafeber HL, Michaelsen KF, Rigo J, Weaver LT: The nutritional and safety assessment of breast milk substitutes and other dietary products for infants: a commentary by the ESPGHAN Committee on Nutrition. J Pediatr Gastroenterol Nutr 2001;32:256–258.
7  Aggett P, Agostoni C, Axelsson I, Goulet O, Hernell O, Koletzko B, Lafeber HN, Michaelsen KF, Morley R, Rigo J, Szajewska H, Weaver LT: Core data for nutrition trials in infants: a discussion document. A commentary by the ESPGHAN Committee on Nutrition. J Pediatr Gastroenterol Nutr 2003;36:338–342.
8  International Conference on Harmonisation of Technical Requirements for Registration of Pharmaceuticals for Human Use. http://www.ich.org. 1996.
9  Handbook Good Laboratory Pratice (GLP). http://www.who.int/tdr/publications/publications/glp-handbook.htm. 2001.
10  Declaration of Helsinki – World Medical Association. http://www.wma.net/e/policy/b3.htm. 2000.
11  de Onis M, Garza C, Onyango AW, Martorell R: WHO Child Growth Standards. Acta Paediatr Suppl 2006;450:5–101.
12  Nelson SE, Rogers RR, Ziegler EE, Fomon SJ: Gain in weight and length during early infancy. Early Hum Dev 1989;19:223–239.

Rose K, van den Anker JN (eds): Guide to Paediatric Clinical Research.
Basel, Karger, 2007, pp 133–134

······················

# Conclusions: Paediatric Drug Development in a Global Context

*Samuel Maldonado*[a]    *John N. van den Anker*[b]    *Klaus Rose*[c]

[a]Women's Health, Wyeth Research, Collegeville, Pa., USA; [b]Division of
Pediatric Clinical Pharmacology, Children's National Medical Center,
and Departments of Pediatrics, Pharmacology and Physiology,
George Washington University School of Medicine and Health Sciences,
Washington, D.C., USA, and Department of Pediatrics, Erasmus MC –
Sophia Children's Hospital, Rotterdam, The Netherlands; [c]Pediatrics,
F. Hoffmann-La Roche Ltd., Pharmaceuticals Division, Basel, Switzerland

As Europe and the United States of America (USA) move forward
with their paediatric initiatives, it is expected that the future of paediatric drug development will be even brighter than in the decade since the
first US paediatric legislation was introduced.

Regarding the mandatory part of paediatric assessment/evaluation
of newly developed drugs, it would be desirable to harmonise the requirements across all regions of the world, as far as possible. Fortunately, an international framework for this harmonisation already exists
with the International Conference on Harmonisation of Technical Requirements for Registration of Pharmaceuticals for Human Use (ICH,
www.ich.org), which now comprises members such as the USA, EU and
Japan, with additional regions and countries as observers. Regional differences due to different ethnic factors are addressed in ICH E 5. Of
course, cultural differences and different medical traditions will continue to exist in different world areas and will continue to influence how
specific drugs are developed. Therefore, the expectations in the drug-
regulatory bodies in the world may not always be the same. However, for

drug development in the paediatric population it would be desirable to create mechanisms to avoid duplicity of efforts given the vulnerability, relative scarcity of subjects, and ethical concerns inherent to this population. This harmonisation should facilitate the timely execution of paediatric drug development plans by the pharmaceutical industry. This paediatric drug development plan should serve the needs of all regulatory bodies simultaneously.

Incentives have proven more successful than any intervention in the past was able to achieve. It would be desirable to make these incentives permanent part of the US law in the USA. Once introduced in Europe, they should remain. The challenge of a global harmonisation of incentives is more difficult to assess. The FDA has issued Written Requests for most modern drugs until now, and the respective research is concluded or underway. For Europe to add a genuine contribution to the use of these medicines in children, pharmaceutical companies will have to propose additional research projects to justify an added European 6 months' market exclusivity. This would constitute a second wave of paediatric research after the first US-triggered one. Should Japan eventually develop significant measures to further facilitate paediatric research, this would then constitute a third wave. An element of competition between the main regions and their regulatory authorities might further advance paediatric research on a worldwide scale.

There is a shared responsibility for all regions of this world, and for both mandatory and voluntary paediatric development between regulatory authorities, health professionals, clinical research, patient advocacy groups and pharmaceutical industry. There will always be open questions and differences of opinion. For the sake of our children's health, the dialogue between these partners in health care should be continued and intensified.

# Subject Index